Star Foods

Selecting a winning team of foods for great health

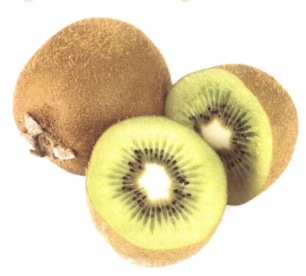

Dr Joanna McMillan Price &
'The Food Coach' Judy Davie

Joanna McMillan Price is a certified nutritionist and dietitian with a PhD in nutritional science from the University of Sydney. She is a popular media spokesperson with regular appearances on TV and radio, and is the nutrition expert for the *Today* show (Nine Network). Joanna has authored/co-authored several previous books including *Reality Food*, *The Low GI Diet* and *The Low GI Diet Cookbook*, she is a health writer for the magazine *Life etc* and writes a regular column 'Ask the food doctor' in *Slimming & Health* magazine. A popular nutrition presenter, Joanna lectures regularly to GPs, practice nurses, fitness instructors and the general public. Originally from Scotland, Joanna emigrated to Australia in 1999 and now lives in Sydney with husband Michael, sons Oliver and Lewis, and Standard Schnauzer, Tosca. You can find Joanna on the net at www.joannamcmillanprice.com.

Judy Davie is a nutrition and food writer and the author of *The Food Coach* (Penguin) and *Read the Label* (Random House). After studies in psychology, food as medicine and macrobiotic cooking she identified a gap in the market beyond what was offered by nutritionists and dietitians and started her own business, The Food Coach, a personal training service in healthy eating. Combining her talents in the kitchen with nutritious food, Judy has written a popular weekly recipe section in *The Sunday Telegraph* and currently has a healthy food guide on www.womansday.com.au. She continues to develop recipes and also writes a column for *Everyday Food* (ACP) and *Healthy Life*. Visit Judy on her popular website www.thefoodcoach.com.au – a source of over 800 healthy recipes and numerous articles and tips on healthy eating and wellbeing.

First published by ABC Books for the
AUSTRALIAN BROADCASTING CORPORATION
GPO Box 9994 Sydney NSW 2001

First published in April 2008

All rights reserved. No part of this publication may be reproduced, stored in a retrieval system or transmitted in any form or by any means, electronic, mechanical, photocopying, recording or otherwise, without the prior written permission of the Australian Broadcasting Corporation.

The National Library of Australia Cataloguing-in-Publication entry
McMillan, Joanna, 1972-
Star foods : selecting a winning team for great health / authors, Dr Joanna McMillan; Judy Davie.

ISBN: 978 0 73332 3386 (pbk.)

1. Nutrition - Popular works. 2. Cookery. I. Davie, Judy, 1962-

613.2

Photography: Still life images by Alfonso Calero Photography www.alfonsocalero.com
Recipe images by John Paul Urizar Photography www.johnpaulurizar.com.au
Cover and internal design and layout by by Leigh Ashforth @ watershed art + design
Indexing by Jon Jermey @ www.webindexing.biz/
Colour reproduction: PageSet, Victoria
Printed by Quality Printing, Hong Kong, China

Contents

Introduction		5
Chapter 1	The Big Picture — Rethinking the Food Pyramid	10
Chapter 2	Vegetables and Fruit	16
Chapter 3	Carbohydrates	52
Chapter 4	Protein	78
Chapter 5	Fats	104
Chapter 6	Drinks	126
Chapter 7	Treats	134
Chapter 8	What's Wrong with Most Diets?	139
Chapter 9	Cooking and Recipes	142
References		219
Index		221

Star Foods

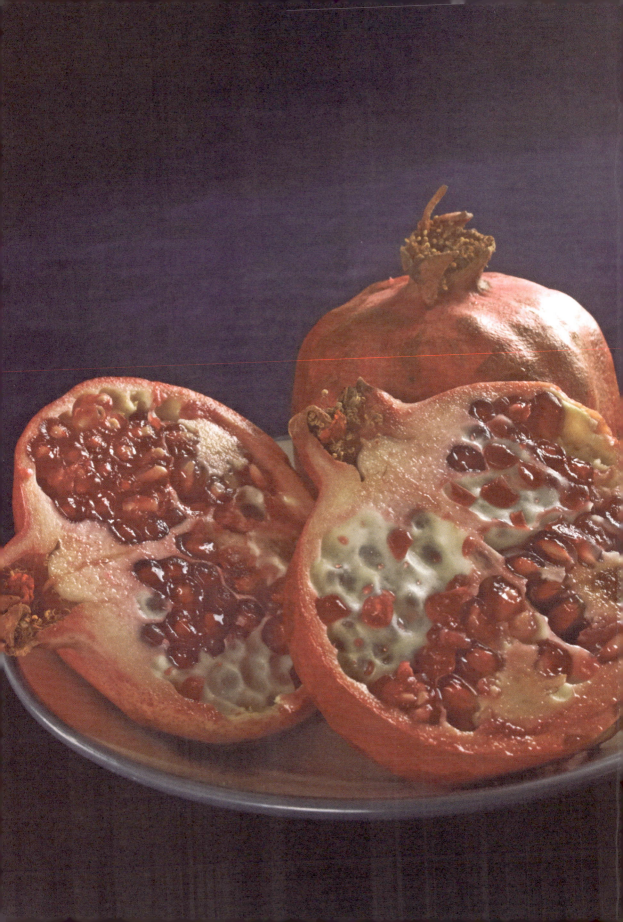

Introduction

What you eat has the power to influence the way you look, how you feel, how much energy you have, your ability to perform mental tasks, your ability to exercise, and your general state of happiness—and that's before we even start to talk about lowering the risk of chronic disease.

Changing to a healthier diet is about being proactive and responsible for your own health and vitality. It's about preventing disease rather than contributing to it. If you speak to anyone who's given up smoking only to start again weeks/months or years later, the chances are they'll tell you that somewhere in the back of their minds they believed they would smoke again. Likewise, anyone who goes 'on a diet' expects to resume their normal eating habits as soon as the diet is over. That is not what this book is about.

The word 'diet' has been misused for too long. It is associated with weight loss and conjures up feelings of guilt, deprivation and misery. But what 'diet' really means, quite simply, is the food you eat on a day-to-day basis. It is our diet that has an impact on our health and wellbeing, and not individual foods or whole food groups. And while disease is influenced by many factors out of our control (genetics being the most obvious example), diet plays an enormous role and is an area we can control.

To be healthy, change your eating habits forever

To be healthy, you have to change your eating habits forever. These are words many of us don't want to hear but they speak the truth. Whether you like it or not, if you want to be healthy and free from the roller-coaster of diet-related mental purgatory, you have no choice but to retrain your eating habits, improve your culinary skills and educate your children to do the same.

The difficulty is in knowing what changes you should make. Who do you believe when barely a day goes by without mention of health scares, obesity problems and miracle cures or concerns about single foods—all information that is usually superseded by something else? It's ludicrous to expect a single food to cure cancer, prevent heart disease, or manage diabetes, and similarly unfair to label any single food as the cause of disease or weight gain. Tomatoes alone won't prevent cancer, nor will a few sweet foods give you diabetes. A sirloin steak won't give you colon cancer, and a potato now and again won't make you fat, even if it is fried. But neither is it fair to categorise entire food groups as good or bad. History has, time and again, shown us that extreme diets eliminating entire food groups inevitably lead to unhealthy attitudes to food, weight problems and poor health. Just as importantly, they're particularly unpalatable, hard to sustain, unsociable and just not fun.

While the science of nutrition gets incredibly complicated as it battles out the intricacies of how foods and drinks affect our health, the conclusions in broader terms are really quite simple and clear.

> *A fresh natural diet including a large variety of minimally processed foods, encompassing every food group, is the safest and healthiest way to eat.*

The organic debate

Some people believe that unless it's 100 per cent organic, from the producer direct to the customer, it's not healthy. Others want the convenience of packaged foods and rely on scientific-sounding supplements to fill any gaps. We take the middle ground. If you want to go organic, that's great. Organic farming helps to protect our planet in a number of ways, not least by reducing the number of chemicals in the air and earth. While there is ongoing scientific debate over the nutritional differences between organic and conventional produce, a European study headed by Newcastle University (UK) has just released findings to show significantly higher levels of particular nutrients, including antioxidants, in organic produce. For example they found the levels of antioxidants in organic milk were up to 90 per cent higher than conventional milk and up to 40 per cent more antioxidants were found in organic vegetables. With this building nutritional evidence and the growing concern over our environment there is no question that buying organic is the ideal. However, the fact is the substantial price hike from conventional to organic means choosing the latter is simply not achievable for many. We hope in time this situation changes, in the meantime what we do know is that fresh produce, eaten (or frozen) within as short a timeframe as possible, does contain more nutrients, whether it is organic or not. You may also want to consider the environmental implications of fossil fuels burned to transport organic 'health foods' from the other side of the world. We therefore recommend eating locally grown food in season as much as possible — if you can afford to support our organic farmers, even better.

Unfortunately, the organic label has also become a bit of a marketing ploy. For example, a processed breakfast cereal remains a processed breakfast cereal—the fact that it is made from organic ingredients doesn't really make it any better for us. Be careful not to assume a product is healthy just because it is organic. (That said, organic products don't contain artificial preservatives, additives or colours and this is certainly advantageous.)

The bottom line is there is much that you can do to improve your diet and your health that will have a far bigger impact than making the leap to organics. There is little point in spending the extra on organics if you continue to smoke socially on the weekend, continue to eat too few plant foods and too many packaged foods, or spend too many hours sitting on your bottom.

Put organics into perspective. Think of a ladder of dietary changes you could make to improve your health with organics right at the top. You can choose to take that final step and eat nothing but organic and manage your life around that ideal, or come down a few notches and simply make the best choices that you can. Certainly climb as high as you can, but not to the point where you're likely to fall. Only make changes that you can reasonably keep up forevermore. This makes it easier, do-able and sustainable.

About this book

This book pulls together scientific facts, assumptions and practical applications. It brings you the latest information from research in the field of nutritional science, while recognising that there's still a lot we don't know. To this end, our ranking of foods is based on fact as far as is possible, but by necessity we have often had to make an educated decision based on the balance of evidence to date. Our ideas are not intended to be set in stone, but provide you with the skills to create a healthy diet that works with your lifestyle and eating preferences.

Our goal is to guide you towards the foods with the potential to give you more bang for your bite, while steering you away from those that may do more harm than good. To this end, we have ranked foods, based on their merits and/or demerits, and created divisions within each food category. Think of the foods you choose to eat as performers in your healthy eating team. Choosing the best players is your best chance of achieving a winning team and therefore a winning diet. The prize is immediate in the way you will look and feel, and both short and long term in maximising your chances of achieving and maintaining good health.

We know that if you eat a wide range of foods from each food group you'll feel good, but you'll feel fabulous if you select the top ranking players from each food group as often as possible. We truly believe there are many people who don't know how good they could look and feel if only they ate better. Experience this for yourself and we guarantee that over time you will increasingly want to eat more of the foods from the top divisions, and fewer of the foods from the bottom; not because we tell you they are better, but because you feel and look better when you choose to eat this way.

This is not a book about deprivation or banning foods. It's not a book to make you feel guilty when you eat or make you a slave to the kitchen forevermore. Enjoying food is a prerequisite to healthy eating. You need to take pleasure in all aspects of food—from selecting good quality produce, preparing it (albeit quickly most of the time) in delicious ways and savouring your efforts. Without a passion for the process, your dietary changes will be unsustainable and you'll soon revert to old habits. Suspend disbelief, open your mind to believe you can eat healthily, enjoy your food and relish in the numerous health benefits as a result.

In short, our aim is to teach you:

★ **What** to eat—selecting the best of the best, the 'star players'

★ **Why** some foods are better than others—the science behind the food

★ **How** to put it all together with easy, quick, healthy and delicious recipes and tips.

Work with the information in this book to find a diet that makes you feel much better than you do. A diet that gives you more energy than you currently have, that allows you to live a fuller life than you are living, one that you enjoy, that's easy to stick to, and one you feel you can stay on forever.

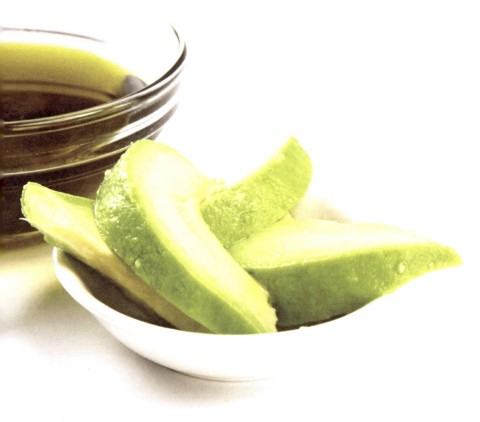

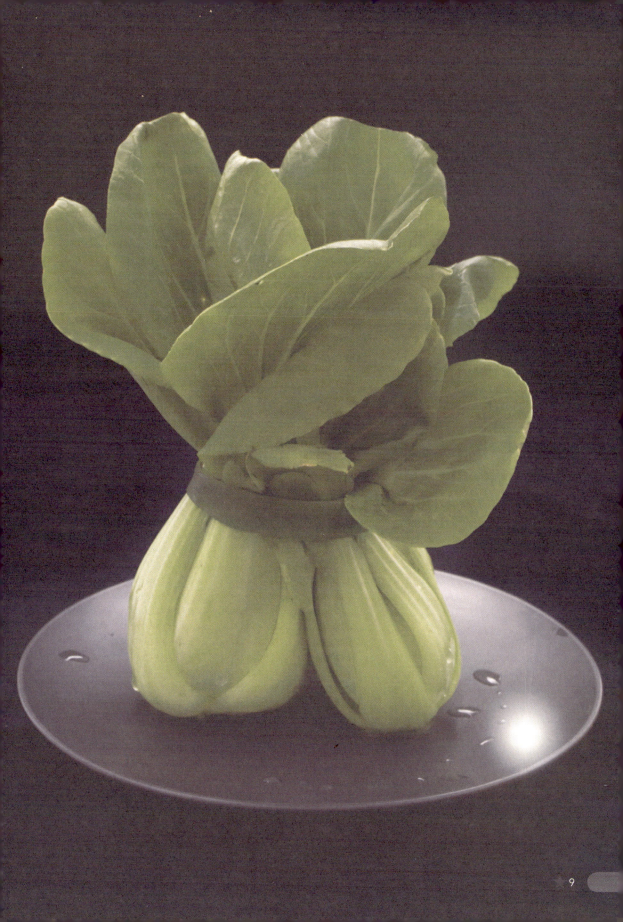

Chapter 1

The Big Picture — Rethinking the Food Pyramid

Before we talk about each food group, it is helpful to think about the role food groups play in our overall diet. This is the big picture and it is good to have it in your head before getting down to the best individual food choices.

You'll notice that our food pyramid in Figure 1.1 differs from the traditional food pyramid. Old-school thinking placed the carbohydrate-rich grain foods — such as bread, rice and pasta — along with vegetables and fruit, at the base. This was intended to encourage us towards a low-fat, high-carbohydrate diet. Yet, as the obesity epidemic threatens to engulf us, this pyramid is failing us fast. While modern diets tend to be energy-dense and nutrient-poor, leading to weight gain and ill health, our revamped food pyramid is designed to reverse this. It will guide you towards a diet that gives you more bang for your bite, a diet that is nutrient dense but energy saving. It is a back-to-nature approach reflecting the way we were designed to eat, and factors in the latest nutrition research.

Vegetables and fruit form the base. For very few kilojoules, vegetables and fruit provide an incredible wealth of essential nutrients. In essence, this means you can afford to eat a lot more of these foods than any other.

On the second level you'll find a flexible line between the more energy-dense, protein-rich and carb-rich foods. So long as you eat the minimum from each group, you can move this line to have more protein and less carbohydrate, or vice versa. How much of each you choose to eat will depend largely on factors such as your food preferences, exercise levels and body type.

Near the top of the pyramid lie the fat-rich foods. Being energy-dense, the volume we eat needs to be less; but because they contain many essential nutrients not found in other foods (not to mention the taste and flavour they impart) they must be included in the daily diet.

And, finally, at the tip of the pyramid are the treats. Treats are the foods and drinks that really give you pleasure but don't add much in the way of nutrients and tend to be loaded with kilojoules. Being energy-dense and nutrient-poor they are the polar opposite of vegetables and fruit at the base of the pyramid.

Examples include chocolate, lollies, a burger, G and T, or whatever else you feel you couldn't live without, regardless of what we say. And neither should you have to. As long as you remember the positioning of treats in the food pyramid and eat them in that proportion so that the bulk of your diet is packed full of 5-star performing foods, it really doesn't matter much what makes up this small space. That said, we will of course try to guide you towards the healthiest treats possible!

Why do we need to eat from each of these food groups? Well it's quite simply this — each food group provides a different set of nutrients and has a special purpose. Without a share of each, your body cannot perform at its best and, sooner or later, you'll feel the effect. Perhaps you don't eat enough vegetables and fruit, and suffer from more colds and flu than you need to; or you've cut out carbs to try and lose weight and find yourself constipated and unable to concentrate. You may have chosen to cut out meat, can't cook fish and don't understand tofu, but you always feel tired, your spirits are low and you never feel fully sated after meals. Or you may be battling with your weight on a low-fat diet and have dry skin, a foul temper and an unbearable craving for a family block of chocolate. The solution is to eat more different foods, not less. Broaden your palate to include foods from each of our food groups, in the proportions illustrated in the pyramid.

The foods that we eat comprise our team in the game of great health. No one player can achieve success alone — it is the collective power of a strong team that produces results. Figure 1.2 illustrates the role of each food group within the team and the green colour indicates the recruitment of the strongest, most 'talented' dietary players.

The game of great health should be played in the same way you play any other sporting game. Play for pleasure but play well. Understand the rules, train hard and select the best players for your team. In the game of great health, the players on your team are the foods you choose to eat. Fresh vegetables and fruit are your defence against infections and chronic disease. They'll protect you from ill health and help you get on with life. Proteins strengthen and maintain the body, while carbohydrates give you the energy and determination to play until the end of each day, and recharge through sleep each night. Fats are the strategic influence on your game and offer mental and physical support whenever you need it. And when you win, you celebrate with a treat … but remember, no team wins by celebrating for longer than they play!

FIGURE 1.1
A new way of thinking about the food pyramid

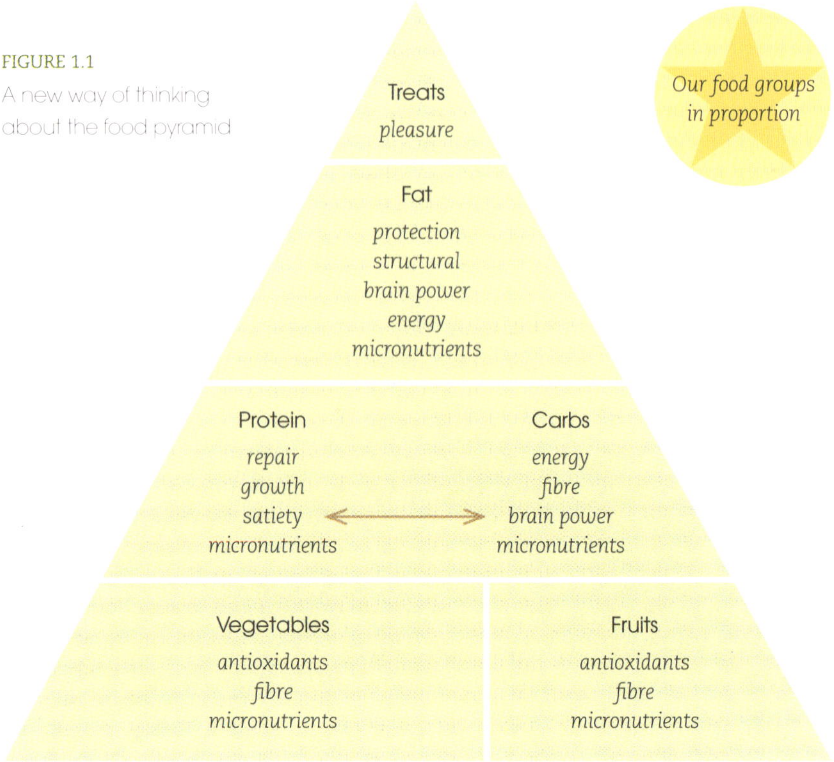

Our food groups in proportion

Treats
pleasure

Fat
protection
structural
brain power
energy
micronutrients

Protein
repair
growth
satiety
micronutrients

Carbs
energy
fibre
brain power
micronutrients

Vegetables
antioxidants
fibre
micronutrients

Fruits
antioxidants
fibre
micronutrients

To help you to select a strong, winning team we rank foods within each of our food groups into five divisions:

★ **5-star performers**—these are the stand-out performers of the team who have that extra flair. These foods give us something extra. Include as many of these in your diet as possible.

★ **Star performers**—consistently good with few flaws, these foods score highly and can happily be included every day.

★ **Good performers**—these are the reliable team members who may lack star qualities but nevertheless have some merit and few flaws.

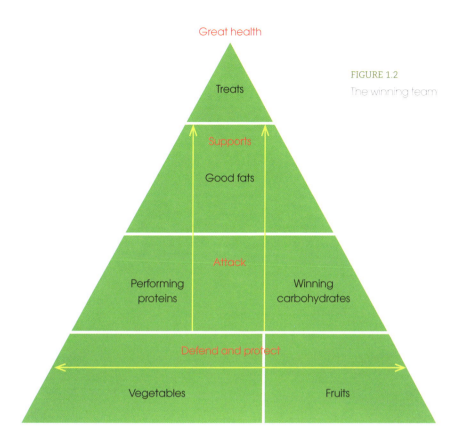

FIGURE 1.2
The winning team

★ Reserves—you wouldn't have these on your team every time but an occasional game is OK. These are the foods with one or more black marks against their name, but some value nevertheless—an 'every now and then' food.

★ Liabilities—if you can avoid them, you would never have these players on your team. These are the foods that have little if anything nutritional to offer, while potentially doing much harm if consumed too often. Make their appearances rare, if at all. However, if they happen to be a food you really, really love, giving them a game *every now and then* will do no harm in the overall scheme of things.

How well are you eating now?

To give yourself an idea about how well you are currently eating, answer our quick quiz. You can then prioritise the changes you need to make to improve your diet. Tick the statements that are true today.

VEGETABLES and FRUIT

- [ ] I eat fewer than five serves of different vegetables a day.
- [ ] I don't eat fresh green leafy vegetables every day.
- [ ] I often eat potatoes or potato products.
- [ ] I eat fewer vegetables than any other food group each day.
- [ ] I eat fewer than two pieces of different fruit each day.
- [ ] I tend to eat the same vegetables and fruit every week.
- [ ] I eat fewer vegetables than fruit.

If you ticked any of the above, your team is likely to be performing below par.
To improve your performance, turn to page 16 and read **Chapter 2: Vegetables and Fruit**.

GRAINS, CEREALS and LEGUMES (carbohydrate-rich foods)

- [ ] I rarely choose foods high in fibre.
- [ ] I am often hungry an hour or two after meals and find it hard not to snack between meals.
- [ ] I regularly eat processed or refined carbohydrates (white breads, crackers, breakfast cereals).
- [ ] I rarely eat legumes and pulses (beans, chickpeas, kidney beans, lentils).
- [ ] I rarely choose wholegrain products.
- [ ] I often avoid carbohydrates to try to lose weight.

If you ticked any of the above, your team is likely to be performing below par.
To improve your performance, turn to page 52 and read **Chapter 3: Carbohydrates**.

MEAT, SEAFOOD, DAIRY, EGGS and LEGUMES (protein-rich foods)

- [ ] I eat fish or seafood less than twice a week.
- [ ] I rarely choose lean cuts of meat and poultry.
- [ ] I don't know how to combine plant foods to meet my protein needs.
- [ ] I rarely choose low-fat dairy products (or soy alternatives).
- [ ] I don't always include a protein source in every meal (from animal or plant).
- [ ] I regularly eat processed meat (salami, pressed cold meats, sausages).

If you ticked any of the above, your team is likely to be performing below par.
To improve your performance, turn to page 78 and read **Chapter 4: Protein**.

OILS, NUTS and SEEDS (fat-rich foods)

- [ ] I eat deep-fried foods more than once a week.
- [ ] I rarely eat nuts and/or seeds.
- [ ] I use butter and/or margarine.
- [ ] I don't know which oils to use for different cooking applications.
- [ ] I eat oily fish less than twice a week.
- [ ] I love fast food and eat it regularly.
- [ ] I usually eat the skin and fat on meat and poultry.

If you ticked any of the above, your team is likely to be performing below par.
To improve your performance turn, to page 104 and read *Chapter 5: Fats*.

DRINKS

- [ ] I drink more than 2 standard drinks a day (standard drink = 100 ml wine, 285 ml full strength beer, 1 nip spirit).
- [ ] I rarely choose to drink plain water.
- [ ] I regularly drink fruit juice and keep cartons in the fridge at home.
- [ ] I drink alcohol almost every night.
- [ ] I often drink coffee or tea but I'm not sure if I should limit my intake of these.
- [ ] I often drink sweetened fizzy drinks or diet drinks on their own or as an alcoholic mixer.

If you ticked any of the above, your team is likely to be performing below par.
To improve your performance, turn to page 126 and read *Chapter 6: Drinks*.

TREATS

- [ ] I eat quite a bit of convenience food (cakes, biscuits, chips, crackers and other snack foods).
- [ ] I eat sweet treats more than three times a week.
- [ ] I often buy confectionery.
- [ ] I often have treats in place of a proper meal.

If you ticked any of the above, your team is likely to be performing below par.
To improve your performance, turn to page 134 and read *Chapter 7: Treats*.

Chapter 2

Vegetables and Fruit

How many times have you heard the message 'eat more fruit and veg'? By now it, no doubt, seems a boring and tired old adage started by your mother and is just a continuing nag to perpetuate with your own kids. But where there is smoke there is fire and, while the world of nutrition science remains controversial about many things, this message has stood the test of time.

The current recommendation in Australia is to eat seven a day (five veggies and two fruit); but the truth is this is almost certainly not the optimum, it's just that this is what is considered achievable given that the vast majority of us fail to even come close to this. You would be hard pressed to find a nutrition expert anywhere in the world who would not agree that one of the most positive things we can do for our health is to up our intake of vegetables and fruit. So think of the seven a day as the minimum and get serious about eating more of these fabulous foods.

Fruit has taken a bit of a bashing following the popularity of low-carb diets and many people believe fruit is bad for them because it contains sugar. Perhaps it is the belief that something that tastes so good cannot possibly be good for us. Thankfully, that is not true as we hope to prove to you in this book. A healthy diet is good for the body, the mind and the taste buds. Sugar in fruit is not the same as foods containing a lot of added refined sugar. The term sugar just means short chain or single carbohydrates—for example, glucose is the type of sugar that circulates in our bloodstream, fructose is found in fruit, lactose is found in milk, and sucrose is the type of sugar we find in packet or table sugar. Sugar is not necessarily bad and, in many cases, is a very good source of energy. The key point is not whether there is sugar present in a food, but whether that sugar is intrinsic to the food (as in the case of fruit and milk) or added to the food (as in many processed foods).

Most fruits have a low glycaemic index (GI) and this means that the sugars present are slowly absorbed, having a smaller and steadier effect on your blood sugar levels than many other foods with little or no sugar present (such as white bread or rice). Fruits are also packed with fibre, antioxidants and other nutrients our bodies need. What's more, humans have eaten fruits (and vegetables) throughout history. It doesn't make sense that low-carb diets exclude these wonderful, naturally sweet foods, while simultaneously promoting the use of processed protein powders and manufactured supplements! We must stop demonising foods based on their carb (or fat) content and look at the bigger picture.

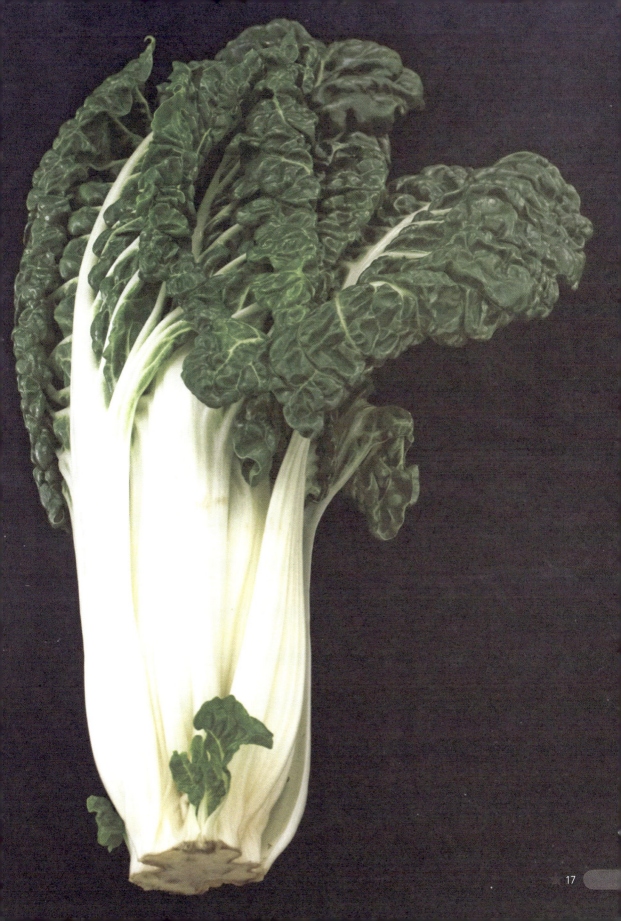

You'll notice we always refer to 'vegetables and fruit' rather than the usual 'fruit and vegetables'. The reason is that we find it far easier to get people eating more fruit as most fruit is sweet and we have an inherent liking for sweet tastes. It tends to be vegetables that are left behind and these are star players in our dietary defence against disease and being overweight. While it's possible to eat more fruit than you really need, it is almost impossible to do the same with vegetables. This is the one food group where you have carte blanche to load your plate and tuck in.

Five reasons for eating more vegetables and fruit

1. Vegetables and fruit are packed with a whole host of **antioxidants** that fight disease and slow the ageing process.
2. Vegetables and fruit provide us with numerous **essential vitamins and minerals** we need to function and perform at our peak.
3. Most vegetables and fruit have a low energy density so, by replacing more energy-dense foods in your diet, they can help with **weight control**.
4. Vegetables and fruit provide **considerable amounts of fibre** and this helps to keep your digestive system healthy, slow blood sugar responses and keep your cholesterol levels in check.
5. Good quality vegetables and fruit **taste delicious!** They add texture, colour, flavour and aroma to dishes when used in the right way.

Ways to eat more

There are many ways to incorporate more vegetables and fruit into your diet. Here are some suggestions to get you started:

- ★ If you can't make it regularly to the grocer or supermarket, use an **online shopping** facility that delivers direct to your door. Many sites now deliver direct from the market, rather than via the major supermarkets, ensuring better quality and freshness.
- ★ Keep the **freezer stocked** with a selection of vegetables including corn cobs, green peas, spinach and stir-fry selection packs. Frozen fruit can also be a great option; for example, frozen berries work well and are often a lot less expensive than the fresh. Freezing preserves the nutrient content and also negates the need for added preservatives.
- ★ **Add vegetables** into dishes such as stews, casseroles, curries and pasta sauces.
- ★ **Stuff sandwiches** and wraps with extra salad fillings.
- ★ Have a **side salad** with your meal whenever possible.
- ★ Keep a **fruit bowl** on your desk and/or at home and grab a piece when you feel hungry between meals or crave something sweet.

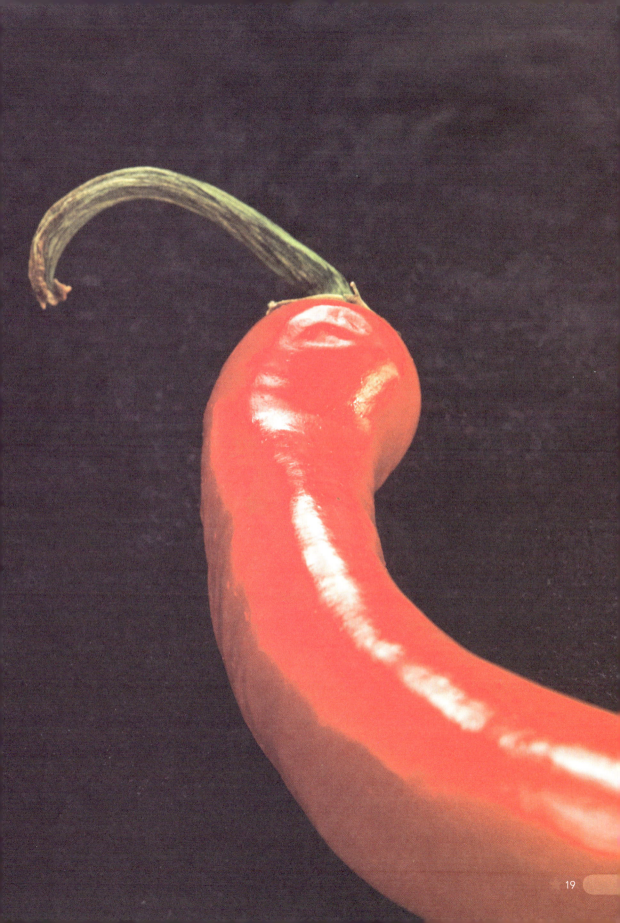

Ranking the Players – Vegetables

Rolling out the vegetable players

Each player was assigned a division based on its nutritional profile. The criteria for the selection process was based on their ability to defend and protect the body and included antioxidant power, fibre content and nutrient density.

	Vegetable	
5-STAR PERFORMERS	asparagus	
	the cabbage family (cruciferous veg/ brassicas)	Asian greens including bok choy, Chinese cabbage and pak choy
		broccoli and broccolini
		Brussels sprouts
		dark green cabbage, for example savoy
		red cabbage
	capsicum and chilli peppers	
	dark green leafy vegetables	curly kale
		endive
		rocket
		silverbeet/Swiss chard
		spinach
		watercress
	globe artichokes	
	mushrooms	
	the onion family (alliums)	garlic
		onions
		leeks
		spring onions
		shallots and eschallots
	parsley	
	peas including green peas and sugar snap/snow peas	
	tomatoes	

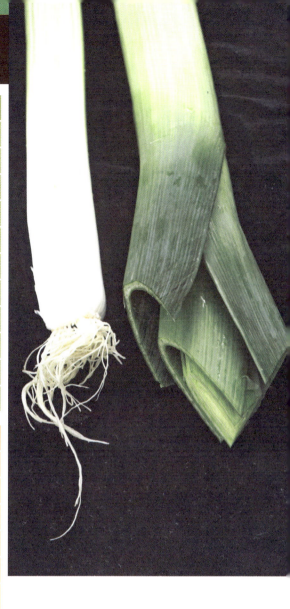

STAR PERFORMERS

Vegetable
carrots
cauliflower
cress, sprouts and bean sprouts
fennel
ginger
green beans, runner beans
green cabbage (pale)
okra
summer squash including zucchini and marrow
sweet potato
winter squash – butternut pumpkin and pumpkin

GOOD PERFORMERS

Vegetable
bamboo shoots
beetroot
celeriac
celery
chicory
cucumber
eggplant
parsnip
radish/white radish (daikons)
small waxy potatoes
taro
turnip/swede
yam

Note: Players are listed alphabetically within each division and not in order of importance.

RESERVES

Vegetable
large floury potatoes

LIABILITIES

Vegetable
none

Vegetables and Fruit ★ 21

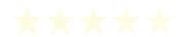

The vegetable 5-star performers Note: In alphabetical order.

ASPARAGUS

In Scotland when we were growing up, asparagus was a rare treat because this wonderful vegetable was hard to come by and it was very expensive. In fact, it was one of the only vegetables to be thought of as a treat and one we all savoured and asked for more. Today, asparagus is far more widely available, although still relatively expensive because of the practicalities involved in growing it in large quantities. It is worth every penny, however. Asparagus is an excellent source of fibre, vitamin A, vitamin C, vitamin K, thiamin, riboflavin, niacin, folate, iron, phosphorus, potassium, copper and manganese. Depending on where it is grown, it can also be an excellent source of the antioxidant mineral selenium. Asparagus also contains:

★ Saponins—compounds thought to prevent heart disease by helping to reduce blood cholesterol levels.

★ Vitamin B6—known for its role in converting food into energy in the body, but this vitamin may also help to reduce PMT and the nausea of early pregnancy. (Be wary of consuming vitamin B6 supplements to treat PMT—too much is toxic and can affect nerve function. Eat your asparagus instead and you can never overdo it!)

★ Rutin—an antioxidant from the bioflavonoid family that plays an important role in strengthening blood vessels. Rutin may therefore be helpful if you have varicose veins, high blood pressure, poor circulation or broken capillaries.

THE CABBAGE FAMILY

Technically called the *Brassica* (genus) or Cruciferous (family) vegetables, the cabbage family includes broccoli, broccolini, cauliflower, Brussels sprouts, bok choy and all varieties of cabbage (dark green cabbages, such as savoy, and red cabbage are particularly nutrient rich). Unfortunately, many of us have been scarred by memories of being forced to eat pale, lifeless, overcooked cabbage or bitter Brussels sprouts and have vowed never to go there again. We hope to convince you otherwise and tempt you back to these fabulous foods.

The cabbage family has been the source of numerous studies after research showed that those who ate the most of these vegetables had lower incidence of some cancers, particularly colon cancer. In fact, one of the first studies Joanna worked on looked at how broccoli affected the susceptibility of cells lining the colon to carcinogenic damage. The findings were that eating raw broccoli provided the most protection for the colon, whereas eating the cooked vegetable got more antioxidants into the bloodstream where they could potentially prevent damage elsewhere in the body (Ratcliffe et al, 2000). In other words, there were different benefits associated with eating the raw and cooked vegetable. You may have assumed eating raw food is always better (many diet books have told us so) but, in fact, the science tells us otherwise. By eating your veggies in both raw and cooked forms, you maximise your body's defences. Raw broccoli florets are deliciously crunchy tossed in a mixed salad, while raw cabbage is a culinary classic in coleslaw and can be fabulously nutritious when prepared in the right way (try Judy's version on page 161 as part of the recipe 'Lentil & Freekeh Patties with Coleslaw'). Broccoli, broccolini and cauliflower all make great additions to a stir-fry, curry or casserole.

The 'Player Profiles' table gives you an overview of the nutrients found in each type of Cruciferous vegetable but, as a family, the key factors are:

A whole host of **phytochemicals** including flavonoids, dithiolthiones, glucosinolates, isothiocyanates, sulforaphane and indoles. Forget about the confusing names, suffice to say that these compounds fight cancer and/or heart disease and probably a whole lot more. We also give you the names as a good illustration of how a supplement antioxidant pill cannot provide nearly the number of goodies found in real food.

Lutein—one of the carotenoid family of antioxidants and is thought to have various benefits for our health. The strongest evidence is for its role in eye health where, along with its partner zeaxanthin, it has been linked to a reduced risk of age-related macular degeneration (AMD), a major cause of vision loss. Lutein may also play a role in maintaining healthy skin, in part by providing some protection against damage from sunlight. At least one study has shown lutein can slow down atherosclerosis (the plaque build-up in the arteries that can eventually cause a heart attack). Finally, lutein is part of the team of antioxidants thought to be important in reducing the risk of certain cancers.

Anthocyanins—the red/purple pigments found in red cabbage. They are powerful antioxidants that contribute to the body's defence against free radical damage.

Insoluble fibre—needed to keep the gut contents moving and prevent constipation.

Folate—a B vitamin of which a good intake can reduce your heart disease risk. If you are planning a baby, folate reduces the risk of neural tube defects.

Vitamin C—one of the key antioxidants and is also important for maintaining a healthy strong immune system. Since vitamin C is easily destroyed in cooking and is lost during storage, aim to include a few raw sources or cook only lightly and eat soon after purchase.

Potassium—important for keeping blood pressure in check.

Vitamin K—for healthy blood-clotting ability. Broccoli and Brussels sprouts are particularly rich in this vitamin.

CAPSICUMS AND CHILLI PEPPERS

Capsicums of all colours and chillies are 5-star performers as they are packed with nutrients that help to protect us from heart disease and cancers as well as being great for eye health. In particular they contain:

★ Beta-carotene—an antioxidant and especially rich in red capsicum. Beta-carotene can also be converted to vitamin A which, among other things, is essential for good vision. Two other carotenoids also important for eye health are lutein and zeaxanthin, found in abundance in red and orange capsicum.

★ Vitamin C—a major antioxidant and, among its many functions, is essential for good immune function and healthy, glowing skin. Since this vitamin is easily destroyed with cooking, try to eat it raw some of the time—for example chop raw capsicum into your salads.

★ Capsaicin—the compound responsible for the heat in chillies. If you like it hot (and the hotter the chilli, the greater the capsaicin content) the good news is that capsaicin has a number of potential benefits; it can ease nasal congestion, encourage cancer-cell death, detoxify cancer-causing compounds and boost your metabolism.

★ Fibre—necessary for good gut function and the soluble fibre can help to reduce blood cholesterol levels. The fibre is found mostly in the skin, however the skin can cause problems for some including those with IBS, diverticulitis or other bowel complaints. If this is the case, grill the capsicum skin side up until blackened, cool and remove the skins. This also sweetens the taste and you can then marinate them and keep them in the refrigerator for a couple of weeks.

DARK GREEN LEAFY VEGETABLES

Another cliché—'eat your greens'! Well, Mum was right again. Dark green leafy vegetables are 5-star performers and the greener the better. While all leaves provide some nutritional value, the dark green leaves found on the likes of kale, silverbeet, Swiss chard, Asian greens, watercress, rocket, spinach, endive and beetroot leaves are especially good. They are packed with nutrients and phytochemicals thought to play essential roles in our health and wellbeing, including:

★ Folate—a B group vitamin important in fighting cancer and heart disease. Low blood folate levels have been associated with an increased risk of heart disease. Since folate is also essential for cell development and DNA replication, a high folate intake prior to conception and in the first three months of pregnancy has been shown to reduce the incidence of birth defects. Endive, spinach and savoy cabbage are particularly good sources.

★ Lutein and zeaxanthin—belong to the carotenoid family of antioxidants and research suggests they are important in keeping your eyes healthy by preventing macular

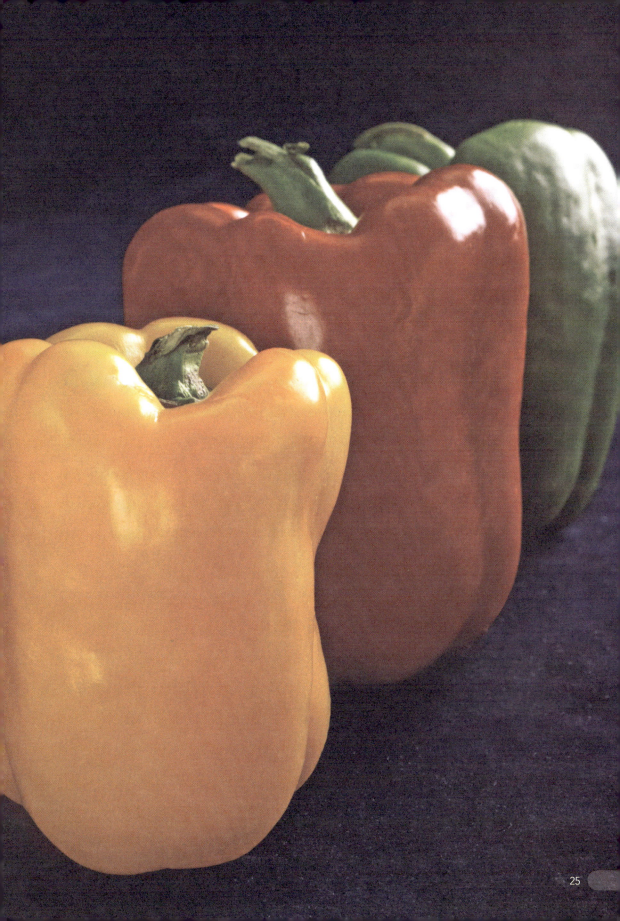

degeneration and possibly cataracts. Kale is an especially abundant source, while spinach, silverbeet, Swiss chard and watercress follow closely behind.

★ Beta-carotene—the most famous carotenoid which gained notoriety from trials linking a high intake to cancer prevention. A similar result was reported from a Finnish trial where again beta-carotene supplements proved detrimental in certain groups (The a-tocopherol b-Carotene Cancer Prevention Study Group, 1994). (More evidence that taking a pill does not have the same effect as consuming a plant-rich diet.) This carotenoid can also be converted to vitamin A in the body when needed, where it then plays an essential role in maintaining good eyesight. Kale again comes top here, but spinach, Swiss chard, silverbeet and all dark greens are not far behind.

> Beware of beta-carotene supplements, however. The infamous CAROT trial had to be stopped after lung cancer incidence actually increased in male smokers and workers exposed to asbestos who were given a supplement containing beta-carotene and vitamin A in combination (Omenn et al, 1996).

★ Vitamin K—a key vitamin in maintaining healthy blood. Kale, watercress, Swiss chard and silverbeet are especially good sources, but all dark green leafy vegetables provide good amounts of this vitamin.

GLOBE ARTICHOKES

Artichokes have been used since ancient times for various medicinal purposes including as a treatment for the liver and there may be a good reason for that—the presence of cynarin (see below). We have to confess that we had almost forgotten this vegetable given that you rarely see it served fresh; it's usually canned or marinated and used in pasta dishes, salads or as a pizza topping. But we discovered that both the leaves and heart of the artichoke have enormous antioxidant capacity and we had to rethink its dietary value. Cooking and using fresh artichokes is a bit of a fiddle but worth having a go as they are delicious and it is the most nutritious way to eat them. Canned artichoke hearts are more convenient and certainly good to have in the pantry, but you do miss out on the many phytonutrients found in the leaves. Key nutrients include:

★ Cynarin—may prevent fat accumulation in the liver and may also promote the production of bile acids required in digestion.

★ The flavonoid luteolin—an antioxidant which seems to be particularly important in preventing damage to LDL-cholesterol, which in turn is involved in the pathogenesis of heart disease. Luteolin may also reduce histamine production and therefore may be of benefit in reducing the inflammation and congestion associated with hayfever and other allergic reactions.

★ Folate—a B group vitamin that we now know is important when you are planning a baby, but is also crucial in preventing cancer and heart disease.

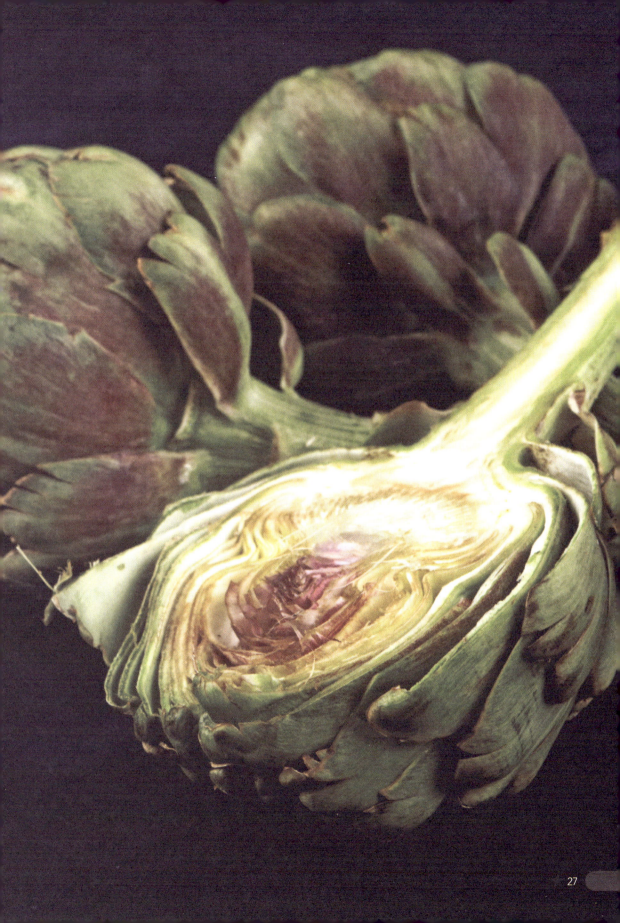

MUSHROOMS

Mushrooms are thought of as a vegetable, but they are actually a fungus with no roots, leaves, flowers or seeds. There are many different varieties and each has a slightly different nutrient profile. Most are a good source of the mineral selenium, often low in modern diets. Selenium has an important antioxidant role and is essential for normal functioning of the thyroid gland. They are also fibre rich and, depending on the variety, are good sources of phosphorus, potassium, copper, manganese and the B group vitamins including folate.

While even the most common forms of mushrooms have many nutritional benefits, it is worthwhile looking for the more unusual varieties such as the Asian mushrooms including shiitake, enoki and maitake, and the large Portobello or flat mushrooms. These have higher levels of particular phytonutrients that may benefit our health. Shiitake mushrooms originated in Asia where they have been consumed and used medicinally for thousands of years. Some of the earliest books on Asian herbal medicine discuss the therapeutic value of the shiitake mushroom. Today, scientific research is uncovering various phytochemicals in shiitakes and other mushrooms that may account for the legendary health benefits. These include:

★ **Lentinan**—a polysaccharide shown to have anti-cancer properties in the laboratory. Studies are ongoing using extracted lentinan with promising results in cancer patients. It also seems to play a role in strengthening the immune system and early studies indicate it may be of value in the treatment of individuals infected with HIV.

★ **Eritadenine**—a compound shown in studies to lower cholesterol in animals.

★ **Ergothioneine**—a powerful antioxidant found in the highest quantities in mushrooms. Wheat germ and chicken liver were previously thought to be the best sources until mushrooms were tested. Shiitake, oyster, king oyster and maitake mushrooms were found to contain as much as 40 times the amount found in wheat germ. The more common button mushrooms can't quite match this, but still contain appreciable amounts and up to 12 times as much as that found in wheat germ (Dubost et al, 2005).

As mushrooms are very porous, it is best not to wash them in water, simply wipe them clean with a damp paper towel. Buy them in a paper bag rather than plastic (this makes them sweat and they will quickly become soggy) and store them in the refrigerator for up to a week. You can also buy mushrooms dried for convenience and most of the nutrients will remain intact. Store these in an airtight container in the refrigerator or freezer where they will stay fresh for as long as a year.

THE ONION FAMILY

The onion family, technically called the *Alliums*, includes not only onions, but leeks, garlic, shallots (sometimes called green onions or even spring onions), spring onions and eschallots (sometimes called French shallots)*. These vegetables seem to be particularly important in preventing cancer of the stomach, but also play a healthy role throughout the gut and in lowering the risk of cardiovascular disease. Unfortunately high-heat cooking destroys some of the disease-fighting nutrients, particularly diallyl sulfide, and we often start a dish by frying the garlic and onion. You might want to try adding them later to a dish or eating them raw on occasion to maximise the health benefit. You may find that raw garlic is not so easy on your digestion; if so, try removing the small green shoot from the middle of the clove before using as this sometimes does the trick.

> * There is confusion over the names of the various onions around the world. In Australia, the most common name given to the long thin green onion with no bulb on the end is a shallot. The long green onion with a white bulb on the end is known as a spring onion and the small dry brown onion with clusters of small bulbs is known as an eschallot.

Some of the key nutrients found in these 5-star performing vegetables are:

★ **Sulphur** compounds—including diallyl sulfide, are shown in research to prevent tumour growth in the stomach, colon and liver. Onions and garlic are particularly good sources.

★ **Antioxidants**—leeks contain kaempferol, which is a flavonoid, red onions quercetin, and don't throw away the green tops of leeks and spring/green onions as these contain the antioxidant carotenoids lutein and zeaxanthin. Both are important for eye health and reduce the risk of age-related macular degeneration and cataracts.

★ Garlic also has **antibacterial** qualities and this may be of benefit in destroying potential harmful bacteria in food and in our gut.

★ **Fructo-oligosaccharides** (FOS)—you have no doubt heard of probiotics (where you consume live beneficial bacteria), well these compounds are prebiotics. They act like fibre in that they pass through the small intestine undigested and enter the colon. There they feed the beneficial bacteria already present, promoting their growth. The by-products of this bacterial fermentation benefit us in many ways including keeping stools soft and easy to pass, keeping the cells lining the colon healthy (preventing cancers) and boosting immune function.

PARSLEY—FLAT LEAF AND CURLY

You might think of parsley as simply a garnish to make a bowl of soup look nice, but that would be to grossly underestimate the herb's nutritional value. Parsley is packed with nutrients including vitamin K, involved primarily in blood clotting, vitamin C, several B group vitamins, useful amounts of iron and other minerals, and the carotenoids beta-carotene, lutein and zeaxanthin. Beta-carotene is an important antioxidant in it's own right, helping to protect the fat-soluble areas of the body, but can also be converted to vitamin A when required. Both lutein and zeaxanthin have been associated with a reduction in the risk of age-related macular degeneration of the eye, a common cause of blindness, and lutein has additionally been shown to play a possible role in preventing colon cancer. Of course one sprig won't do much good, you need to use more of it to gain the benefits. The classic Middle Eastern dish, tabouli is packed with fresh parsley, or you could add liberally at the end of cooking to sauces, soups, casseroles or mix through a salad.

PEAS—GREEN, SUGAR SNAP / SNOW PEAS

By peas we are including green peas (fresh or frozen) and sugar snap/snow peas, which are just a variety of peas that we eat pod and all. All varieties of peas contain a wealth of important nutrients including the carotenoids beta-carotene, alpha-carotene, lutein and zeaxanthin. While all of these have the potential to act as powerful disease-fighting antioxidants, they are also important for eye health. Alpha- and beta-carotene can be converted to vitamin A in the body, a nutrient essential for good vision, while lutein and zeaxanthin are found in abundance in the eye and reduce the risk of age-related macular degeneration. Green peas are particularly rich in lutein and zeaxanthin. All peas are fibre rich and therefore great for your gut. As with other legumes, they are high in soluble fibre that binds to cholesterol in the gut, helping to reduce blood levels. Peas also provide a range of vitamins and minerals—in particular, the antioxidant vitamin C, vitamin K required for healthy blood and strong bones, the B group vitamins necessary for carbohydrate, protein and fat metabolism, and iron for normal blood cell formation and function. Peas do provide a higher carbohydrate level than other vegetables, and therefore slightly more energy but, given that you are highly unlikely to overeat them, this is really not a concern! They do also provide a reasonable amount of plant protein and so are a particularly good inclusion in vegetarian diets.

TOMATOES

We hear lots about the antioxidants vitamins A, C and E and beta-carotene, but we hope you are getting the picture that there are in fact many more antioxidants found in food. Tomatoes are listed among our top veggies because they contain lycopene, an antioxidant that may be even more powerful than vitamin C. Lycopene is found in other red foods, such as pink grapefruit and watermelon, but undoubtedly the best source is tomato and tomato products. In fact, this is an unusual case where food processing actually increases the availability of the nutrient, as shown in Table 2.1.

TABLE 2.1 Lycopene in foods

Product	Lycopene (milligrams / 100 g)	Serving size	Lycopene (milligrams / serving)
Tomato paste	42.2	2 tablespoons	13.8
Pasta sauce	21.9	0.5 cup	28.1
Tomato sauce (ketchup)	14.1	0.25 cup	8.9
Tomato juice	9.5	1 cup	25.0
Pink grapefruit	4.0	0.5 fruit	4.9
Raw tomato	3.0	1 medium	3.7

From Table 2.1, you can see that tomato paste is fabulously rich in lycopene, especially when compared to a raw tomato. As we eat a greater quantity of pasta sauce and tomato juice, these foods provide the most lycopene per serve. Try adding tomato paste into soups, sauces and casseroles; add a dash of Worcestershire sauce and Tabasco to tomato juice for a spicy refreshing drink; or try our recipe for Basic Tomato and Basil Sauce on page 173. While there is no consensus yet on how much we need, the best studies from Harvard (Giovannucci 1999) suggest we should be eating one or two tomato products every day.

But, it's not all about **lycopene**, other goodies in tomatoes include:

★ Beta-carotene—a potent antioxidant linked to reduced cancer risk when consumed in foods (infamously not so when consumed as a supplement where it can actually increase cancer growth rate, see page 24 under dark green leafy vegetables).

★ **Caffeic** and **ferulic acids**—involved in the production of cancer-fighting enzymes in the body.

★ **Chlorogenic acid**—believed to help detoxify carcinogens and viruses.

★ **Lutein** and **zeaxanthin**—the carotenoids we have met several times already, thought to be important in preventing eye disease.

Player Profiles – Vegetables

5-STAR PERFORMERS

Vegetable		Nutrient Summary
asparagus		Very good source of dietary fibre, vitamin C, vitamin E, vitamin K, thiamin, riboflavin, niacin, vitamin B6, folate, iron, phosphorus, potassium, copper and manganese. Good source of the antioxidant beta-carotene, which can also be converted to vitamin A in the body; and in two other carotenoid antioxidants, lutein and zeaxanthin. These promote eye health, reducing the risk of age-related macular degeneration and cataracts. Lutein may also play a role in preventing colon cancer. Good source of vitamin B5, calcium, magnesium, zinc and selenium. Contains saponins—thought to reduce cholesterol levels and reduce heart disease risk—and rutin, an antioxidant involved in strengthening blood vessels.
the cabbage family (cruciferous veg/brassicas)	Asian greens including bok choy, Chinese cabbage and pak choy	Extremely rich in the antioxidant beta-carotene, which can also be converted to vitamin A in the body. Very good source of vitamin C, vitamin K, riboflavin, vitamin B6, folate, calcium, iron, magnesium, potassium and manganese. Good source of dietary fibre, thiamin, niacin and phosphorus.
	broccoli and broccolini	Rich in the antioxidant carotenoids lutein and zeaxanthin, which promote eye health, reducing the risk of age-related macular degeneration and cataracts. Lutein may also play a role in preventing colon cancer. Good source of the antioxidant beta-carotene, which can also be converted to vitamin A in the body. Very good source of dietary fibre, vitamin C, vitamin K, vitamin B6, folate, potassium and manganese. Good source of vitamin E, thiamin, riboflavin, vitamin B5, calcium, iron, magnesium, phosphorus and selenium.
	Brussels sprouts	Rich in the antioxidant carotenoids lutein and zeaxanthin, which promote eye health, reducing the risk of age-related macular degeneration and cataracts. Lutein may also play a role in preventing colon cancer. Good source of the antioxidant beta-carotene, which can also be converted to vitamin A in the body. Very good source of dietary fibre, vitamin C, vitamin K, thiamin, vitamin B6, folate, potassium and manganese. Good source of riboflavin, iron, magnesium and phosphorus.
	dark green cabbage, for example savoy	Very good source of dietary fibre, vitamin C, vitamin K, vitamin B6, folate, magnesium, potassium, manganese and the antioxidant beta-carotene, which can be converted to vitamin A in the body. Good source of thiamin, calcium, phosphorus and copper.
	red cabbage	Very good source of the antioxidant beta-carotene, which can be converted to vitamin A in the body. Very good source of dietary fibre, vitamin C, vitamin K, vitamin B6, potassium and manganese. Good source of thiamin, riboflavin, folate, calcium, iron and magnesium.
capsicum and chilli peppers		Rich in the antioxidant beta-carotene, which can be converted to vitamin A in the body. Very good source of dietary fibre, vitamin C, vitamin E, vitamin K, vitamin B6, potassium and manganese. Good source of thiamin, riboflavin, niacin, folate, vitamin B5 and magnesium. Provides small amounts of lycopene, a member of the carotenoid family and a powerful antioxidant. Preliminary research suggests lycopene may play a role in the fight against cancer. One of the few food sources of a lesser known carotenoid called beta-cryptoxanthin which may reduce the risk of lung and colon cancer, and rheumatoid arthritis. Chillies can boost your metabolism if you eat enough of them!
dark green leafy vegetables	curly kale	Not always easy to source in Australia but well worth buying when you see it. One of the best sources of the antioxidant carotenoids lutein and zeaxanthin. These promote eye health, reducing the risk of age-related macular degeneration and cataracts. Lutein is also thought to play a role in preventing colon cancer. Also rich in the antioxidant beta-carotene which can also be converted to vitamin A in the body. Very good source of vitamin C, vitamin K, vitamin B6, calcium, potassium, copper and manganese. Good source of dietary fibre, thiamin, riboflavin, folate, iron, magnesium and phosphorus.
	endive	Rich in the antioxidant beta-carotene, which can also be converted to vitamin A in the body. Very good source of dietary fibre, vitamin C, vitamin K, thiamin, riboflavin, folate, vitamin B5, calcium, iron, potassium, zinc, copper and manganese. Good source of vitamin E, magnesium and phosphorus.

Star Foods

The table below summarises the attributes of each of our vegetable players including key nutrients present, the GI where relevant, and any additional information of note.

	Vegetable	Nutrient Summary
dark green leafy vegetables (cont.)	rocket	Rich in the antioxidant beta-carotene, which can also be converted to vitamin A in the body. Also a great source of two other antioxidant carotenoids, lutein and zeaxanthin. These promote eye health, reducing the risk of age-related macular degeneration and cataracts. Lutein is also thought to play a role in preventing colon cancer. Very good source of dietary fibre, vitamin C, vitamin K, folate, calcium, iron, magnesium, phosphorus, potassium and manganese. Also good levels of thiamin, riboflavin, vitamin B6, vitamin B5, zinc and copper.
	silverbeet/ Swiss chard	Extremely rich in the antioxidant carotenoids lutein and zeaxanthin. These promote eye health, reducing the risk of age-related macular degeneration and cataracts. Lutein is also thought to play a role in preventing colon cancer. Also a fabulous source of the better known carotenoid, beta-carotene which, in addition to its antioxidant potential, can be converted to vitamin A in the body. Very good source of dietary fibre, vitamin C, vitamin E, vitamin K, riboflavin, vitamin B6, calcium, iron, magnesium, phosphorus, potassium, copper and manganese. Good source of thiamin, folate and zinc.
	spinach	Extremely rich in the antioxidant carotenoids lutein and zeaxanthin. These promote eye health, reducing the risk of age-related macular degeneration and cataracts. Lutein is also thought to play a role in preventing colon cancer. Also a fabulous source of the better known carotenoid, beta-carotene which, in addition to its antioxidant potential, can be converted to vitamin A in the body. Very good source of dietary fibre, vitamin C, vitamin E, vitamin K, vitamin B6, thiamin, riboflavin, folate, calcium, iron, magnesium, phosphorus, potassium, copper and manganese. Good source of niacin and zinc.
	watercress	Great source of the antioxidant carotenoids lutein, zeaxanthin and beta-carotene. The first two promote eye health, reducing the risk of age-related macular degeneration and cataracts. Lutein may also play a role in preventing colon cancer. Beta-carotene, in addition to its antioxidant role, can be converted to vitamin A in the body. Very good source of vitamin C, vitamin E, vitamin K, thiamin, riboflavin, vitamin B6, calcium, magnesium, phosphorus, potassium and manganese. Good source of protein, folate, vitamin B5 and copper.
	globe artichokes	Very good source of dietary fibre, vitamin C, vitamin K, folate, magnesium, copper and manganese. Good source of vitamin B6, iron, phosphorus and potassium. Also contains cynarin, thought to be important for liver health, and the antioxidant luteolin which has anti-inflammatory properties and may be helpful in relieving symptoms of hayfever and other allergic reactions.
	mushrooms	Very good source of vitamin D, thiamin, riboflavin, niacin, vitamin B6, vitamin B5, phosphorus, potassium, copper and selenium. A good source of dietary fibre, protein, vitamin C, folate, iron, zinc and manganese. Shiitake and other Asian varieties seem to be particularly rich in additional phytochemicals that may provide defence against cancer and other chronic diseases.
the onion family (alliums)	garlic, onions, leeks, spring onions, shallots and eschallots	Very good source of dietary fibre, vitamin C, vitamin K, folate, calcium, iron, potassium and manganese and a good source of thiamin, riboflavin, magnesium, phosphorus and copper. Contain disease-fighting nutrients, including sulphur compounds and antioxidants thought to be important in preventing cancer and heart disease. Shallots, spring onions and leeks are the more nutrient-dense, while garlic has antibacterial properties. Onions and eschallots contain fructo-oligosaccharides (FOS) that encourage the growth of beneficial bacteria in the colon.
	parsley	Extremely rich in the antioxidant beta-carotene, which can also be converted to vitamin A in the body. Good source of two other antioxidant carotenoids, lutein and zeaxanthin. These promote eye health, reducing the risk of age-related macular degeneration and cataracts. Lutein may also play a role in preventing colon cancer. Very good source of dietary fibre, vitamin C, vitamin K, folate, calcium, iron, magnesium, potassium, copper and manganese. Good source of vitamin E, thiamin, riboflavin, niacin, vitamin B6, vitamin B5, phosphorus and zinc.
	peas including green peas and sugar snap/snow peas	Good source of the antioxidant carotenoids lutein and zeaxanthin. These promote eye health, reducing the risk of age-related macular degeneration and cataracts. Lutein may also play a role in preventing colon cancer. Smaller but useful levels of the more familiar antioxidant carotenoid beta-carotene that can be converted to vitamin A in the body. A very good source of dietary fibre, vitamin C, vitamin K, thiamin, folate, iron and manganese. A good source of riboflavin, vitamin B6, vitamin B5, magnesium, phosphorus and potassium.
	tomatoes	Cooked tomatoes and tomato paste are particularly rich sources of lycopene, a carotenoid antioxidant that may be more powerful than vitamin C and shown in preliminary research to provide protection from a number of cancers. Tomatoes also contain lutein and zeaxanthin, beta-carotene, and caffeic, ferulic and chlorogenic acids—all thought to play roles in fighting cancer and other disease. Very good source of dietary fibre, vitamin C, vitamin K, potassium and manganese. Good source of vitamin E, thiamin, niacin, vitamin B6, folate, magnesium, phosphorus and copper.

Player Profiles – Vegetables (continued)

STAR PERFORMERS

Vegetable	Nutrient Summary
carrots	Hard to beat for the antioxidant beta-carotene which can also form vitamin A in the body. Very good source of dietary fibre, vitamin C, vitamin K and potassium. Good source of thiamin, niacin, vitamin B6, folate and manganese.
cauliflower	Very good source of dietary fibre, vitamin C, vitamin K, vitamin B6, folate, vitamin B5, potassium and manganese. Good source of protein, thiamin, riboflavin, niacin, magnesium and phosphorus.
cress, sprouts and bean sprouts	Very good source of vitamin C, vitamin K, riboflavin, vitamin B6, folate, calcium, iron, magnesium, phosphorus, potassium, copper and manganese. A good source of dietary fibre, vitamin E, thiamin and niacin. Cress is extremely rich in the antioxidant carotenoids beta-carotene, lutein and zeaxanthin. The latter two promote good eye health by reducing the risk of age-related macular degeneration and cataracts. Lutein may also be important in preventing colon cancer. Beta-carotene, in addition to its antioxidant role, can be converted to vitamin A in the body.
fennel	Very good source of dietary fibre, vitamin C, folate, potassium and manganese. Also a good source of niacin, calcium, iron, magnesium, phosphorus and copper.
ginger	Can be an effective treatment for nausea, particularly motion sickness. Contains nutrients known to be anti-inflammatory. Early research shows promise for ginger in heart disease prevention by preventing blood clots and lowering cholesterol. Good source of vitamin C, magnesium, potassium, copper and manganese.
green beans, runner beans	Very good source of dietary fibre, vitamin A, vitamin C, vitamin K, folate and manganese. Also a good source of thiamin, riboflavin, niacin, vitamin B6, calcium, iron, magnesium, phosphorus, potassium and copper. Provides good amounts of the antioxidant carotenoids beta-carotene, lutein and zeaxanthin. The latter two promote good eye health by reducing the risk of age-related macular degeneration and cataracts. Lutein may also be important in preventing colon cancer. Beta-carotene, in addition to its antioxidant role, can be converted to vitamin A in the body.
green cabbage (pale)	Very good source of vitamin A, vitamin C, vitamin K, riboflavin, vitamin B6, folate, calcium, iron, magnesium, potassium and manganese. A good source of dietary fibre, protein, thiamin, niacin and phosphorus.
okra	Dietary fibre-rich and a very good source of vitamin C, vitamin K, thiamin, vitamin B6, folate, calcium, magnesium, phosphorus, potassium and manganese. Good source of riboflavin, niacin, iron, zinc and copper.
summer squash including zucchini and marrow	Fibre rich and a very good source of vitamin C, vitamin K, riboflavin, vitamin B6, folate, magnesium, potassium and manganese. Good source of thiamin, niacin, phosphorus and copper.
sweet potato	The orange-coloured varieties are rich in the antioxidant carotenoid beta-carotene, which can also be converted to vitamin A in the body. All varieties provide good amounts of dietary fibre, vitamin B6, potassium and manganese. Australian sweet potatoes (but not the New Zealand kumara) have a low GI making them great for sustained energy and good filling power.
winter squash including butternut pumpkin and pumpkin	Extremely rich in the lesser known antioxidant carotenoid beta-cryptoxanthin, which may reduce the risk of lung and colon cancer as well as rheumatoid arthritis. Rich in beta-carotene which, in addition to its antioxidant role, can be used to form vitamin A in the body. Pumpkin also provides two further antioxidant carotenoids, lutein and zeaxanthin, shown to promote good eye health by reducing the risk of age-related macular degeneration and cataracts. Lutein may also be important in preventing colon cancer. All provide very good levels of vitamin C, potassium, riboflavin and manganese and good amounts of dietary fibre, vitamin E, thiamin, niacin, vitamin B6, folate, calcium and magnesium.

GOOD PERFORMERS

Vegetable	Nutrient Summary
bamboo shoots	Very good source of vitamin B6, potassium, copper and manganese. Good source of dietary fibre, protein, riboflavin and zinc.
beetroot	Very good source of folate and manganese. Good source of dietary fibre, vitamin C, magnesium and potassium. Beet greens are in fact far more nutritious than the root providing an excellent range of essential nutrients.
celeriac	Very good source of vitamin C, vitamin K, phosphorus and potassium. Good source of dietary fibre, vitamin B6, magnesium and manganese.
celery	Very good source of dietary fibre, vitamin C, vitamin K, folate, potassium and manganese. Also provides good levels of a range of carotenoid antioxidants which can form vitamin A in the body.
chicory	Very good source of dietary fibre, vitamin C, thiamin, folate, potassium and manganese. Good source of vitamin B6, magnesium, phosphorus and copper.
cucumber	Provides good levels of vitamin K and vitamin C, and small amounts of various minerals.
eggplant	Dietary fibre-rich and a very good source of folate, potassium and manganese. Good source of vitamin C, vitamin K, thiamin, niacin, vitamin B6, vitamin B5, magnesium, phosphorus and copper.
parsnip	Very good source of dietary fibre, vitamin C, vitamin K, folate and manganese. Good source of potassium. Parsnips do have a high GI but you can ignore this since they have very little carbohydrate in a usual serving.
radish/white radish (daikons)	Fibre-rich and a good source of vitamin C, folate, potassium, riboflavin, vitamin B6, calcium, magnesium, copper and manganese. White radish or daikons are the Asian variety.
small waxy potatoes	These have a lower GI than large floury potatoes and are therefore a better choice. However, aside from providing carbohydrate energy, potatoes are not particularly nutrient rich. They do provide good levels of vitamin C, but this is easily destroyed during storage and cooking. The skin is more nutrient-rich than the flesh providing good levels of fibre, vitamin B6 and potassium.
taro	Not so popular in Australia but a staple in many tropical regions of the world. A starchy vegetable that has a low GI providing a slow-burning energy source. Good source of dietary fibre, vitamin E, vitamin B6, potassium and manganese. The leaves can also be eaten and are highly nutritious if you can find them.
turnip/swede	Fibre-rich and provides reasonable levels of vitamin C, manganese, vitamin B6, folate, calcium, potassium and copper.
yam	High in carbohydrate but also low GI and is therefore filling and provides long-lasting energy. Very good source of vitamin C. Good source of dietary fibre, vitamin B6, potassium and manganese.

RESERVES

large floury potatoes	Very high GI and easy to overeat in all forms. These types of potatoes have been bred for a bland taste, white colour and large size. As a result, they are far removed from the original plant form and are unfortunately far less nutritious. Some vitamin C and good carb source for recovery after strenuous exercise. For most, however, there are far more nutritious choices to be had.

LIABILITIES

none	All veggies have something to offer us and the only liability would be in how they were handled; for example, deep-frying, overcooking and processing.

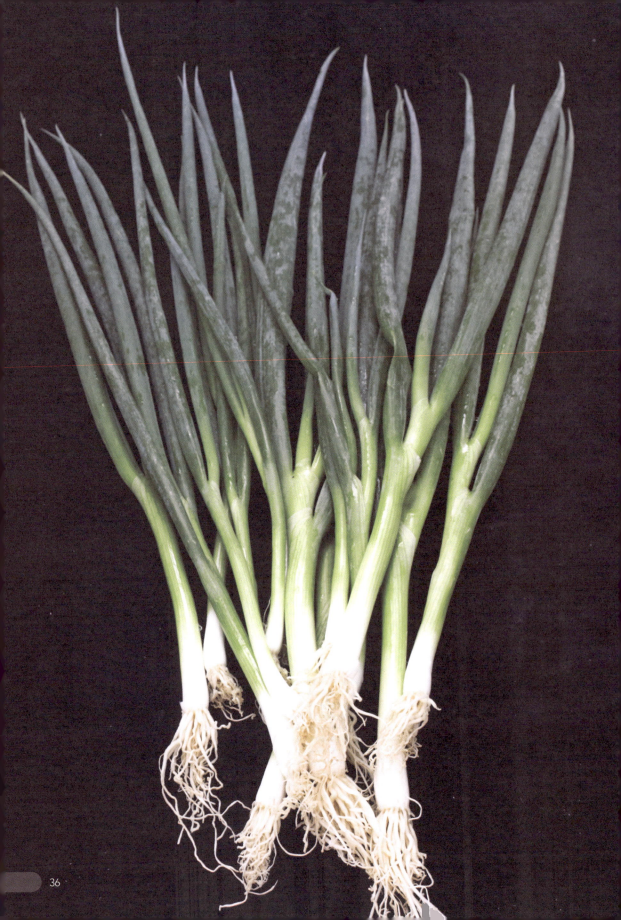

Ranking the Players – Fruit

Rolling out the fruit players

Each player was assigned a division based on its nutritional profile. The criteria for the selection process were based on their ability to defend and protect the body and included antioxidant power, fibre content, GI and nutrient density. Consideration was also given to added sugar and other additives used in processing.

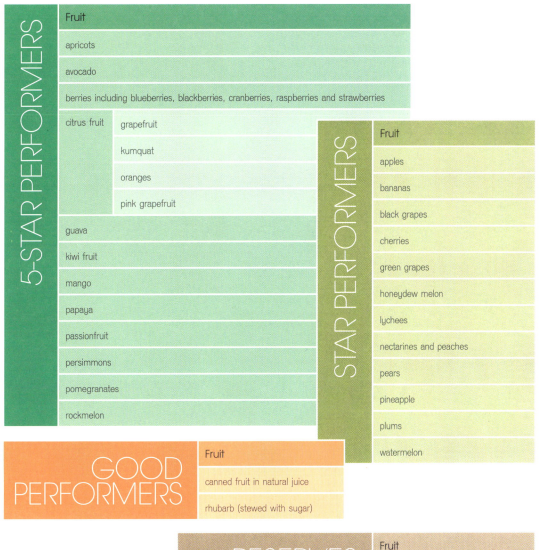

5-STAR PERFORMERS

Fruit
apricots
avocado
berries including blueberries, blackberries, cranberries, raspberries and strawberries
citrus fruit — grapefruit, kumquat, oranges, pink grapefruit
guava
kiwi fruit
mango
papaya
passionfruit
persimmons
pomegranates
rockmelon

STAR PERFORMERS

Fruit
apples
bananas
black grapes
cherries
green grapes
honeydew melon
lychees
nectarines and peaches
pears
pineapple
plums
watermelon

GOOD PERFORMERS

Fruit
canned fruit in natural juice
rhubarb (stewed with sugar)

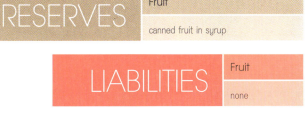

RESERVES

Fruit
canned fruit in syrup

LIABILITIES

Fruit
none

Note: Frozen fruit is usually just as nutritious as fresh—sometimes more so as nutrients easily lost in storage or with exposure to light, such as vitamin C, are preserved. Furthermore, freezing is itself a preservative meaning that artificial preservatives need not be added.

Ranking the Players – Dried Fruit

5-STAR PERFORMERS

Dried Fruit
apricots
prunes

Note: The drying process results in a loss of some nutrients found in fresh fruit and are more energy dense than fresh which is why they fall into the good performing category rather than star. Prunes and apricots provide exceptional other quality benefits and are rated 5-star performers accordingly.

GOOD PERFORMERS

Dried Fruit
apple
currents
dates
figs
mango
peach
pear
raisins
sultanas

RESERVES

Dried Fruit
cranberries (raisins)

LIABILITIES

Dried Fruit
none

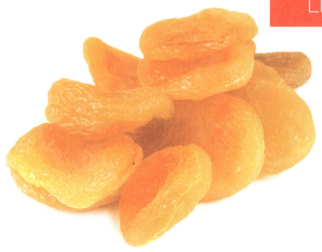

Note: Preservatives such as sulphites are often used in the processing of dried fruits. Those with asthma, especially children, may be particularly sensitive and should avoid this preservative. Look for preservative-free or organic produce to avoid this.

The fruit 5-star performers Note: In alphabetical order.

APRICOTS, FRESH AND DRIED

The wonderful orange colour comes from the carotenoids present in apricots. They are particularly high in the potent antioxidant beta-carotene. Only three apricots provide about half of the daily amount of beta-carotene experts recommend. Beta-carotene is believed to play a role in preventing damage to cells from free radicals that lead to heart disease, cancers and accelerated ageing. It can also be converted to vitamin A, essential for good vision, when intakes of this vitamin are insufficient. Fresh apricots are also good sources of vitamin C, adding to the antioxidant power of the fruit as well as being essential for a strong immune function and healthy skin. Drying the fruit unfortunately destroys much of the vitamin C, but most of the other nutrients are preserved and are, indeed, concentrated in this form. Dried apricots of course have a higher energy density so, if you are watching your weight, you can't eat unlimited amounts. However, they do have a low GI and make a great between-meal snack. The dried fruit is particularly good for iron, essential for the production of properly functioning red blood cells, and is also a good laxative.

AVOCADO

The days of the low-fat dogma have cast a shadow on the poor avocado, yet it has so much to offer us. Yes it does indeed contain a lot of fat, so you can't eat it until the cows come home, but you are unlikely to given its rich flavour. The fat in avocados is predominately unsaturated, mostly monounsaturated like that found in olive oil. This makes it an ideal replacement for butter on bread and you can buy avocado oil for cooking and to use in salad dressings. This type of fat not only has benefits on our cholesterol levels and in reducing cardiovascular disease risk, it also seems to be more easily burnt as fuel rather than being deposited on our hips—all good news if you are battling with weight control. Not only that, but avocados also give us:

★ **Vitamin E**—the major fat-soluble antioxidant that protects the fatty outer layers of cells from free radical damage.

★ **Vitamin C**—a water-soluble antioxidant that strengthens the immune system, and also recycles vitamin E keeping it functioning. This is an example of how no nutrient works in isolation but as a team effort.

★ **Folate**—essential for women planning a baby, but also in preventing heart disease by lowering homocysteine levels in the blood and in reducing the risk of cancer as folate is key in the production of DNA and new cells.

★ **Fibre**—half an avocado provides 6–7 grams of fibre, putting you well on your way to meeting your daily target of 25–30 grams.

- ⭐ **Vitamin K**—plays an essential role in blood clotting.
- ⭐ **Glutathione**—an antioxidant involved in preventing free radical damage to cells.
- ⭐ **Potassium** and **magnesium**—both may help keep blood pressure down. Magnesium can also help migraine sufferers and reduce symptoms of PMT.
- ⭐ **Beta-sitosterol**—a compound currently being studied for its potential to prevent breast cancer. It may also reduce the symptoms of prostate enlargement (benign prostatic hyperplasia or BPH) that often plagues men as they get older.

BERRIES

Berries look and taste delectable, so it seems too good to be true that they can actually be good for us. Yet berries come top of the tree when it comes to comparing the antioxidant power of all plant foods and they are packed with other nutrients our bodies need.

Key nutrients found in berries include:

- ⭐ **Anthocyanins**—a sub-group of the flavonoids and responsible for the purple/red colour of berries; these are powerful antioxidant compounds.
- ⭐ **Ellagic acid**—particularly rich in strawberries, raspberries and blackberries and seems to have anti-cancer properties. In laboratory experiments it has been shown to induce cancer-cell death and act as an antioxidant (Han et al, 2006).
- ⭐ **Kaempferol**—yet another antioxidant which may also reduce LDL-cholesterol.
- ⭐ **Tannins**—can prevent bacteria from attaching to the urinary tract and thus are useful in staving off cystitis (found in cranberries, blackberries and blueberries).
- ⭐ **Vitamin C**—strawberries and fresh cranberries are particularly rich, it is important in maintaining a strong immune system and, is essential in the production of collagen. Healthy skin therefore relies on a good vitamin C intake.

CITRUS FRUIT

Unfortunately, for many people, drinking orange juice is the closest they come to enjoying the benefits of citrus fruit. This group includes oranges of all varieties, tangerines, mandarins, clementines, grapefruit, pink grapefruit, lemons and limes. Vitamin C probably comes to mind as the key nutrient and, indeed, a single orange provides about one-and-a-half times your daily requirement (and we suspect more may be beneficial). Many of us reach for vitamin C supplements when we have a cold or flu and we may be right to do so. A recent review of the evidence concluded that, while vitamin C does not seem to stop you catching the cold, it is indeed involved in respiratory defences and has (an albeit small) benefit on reducing

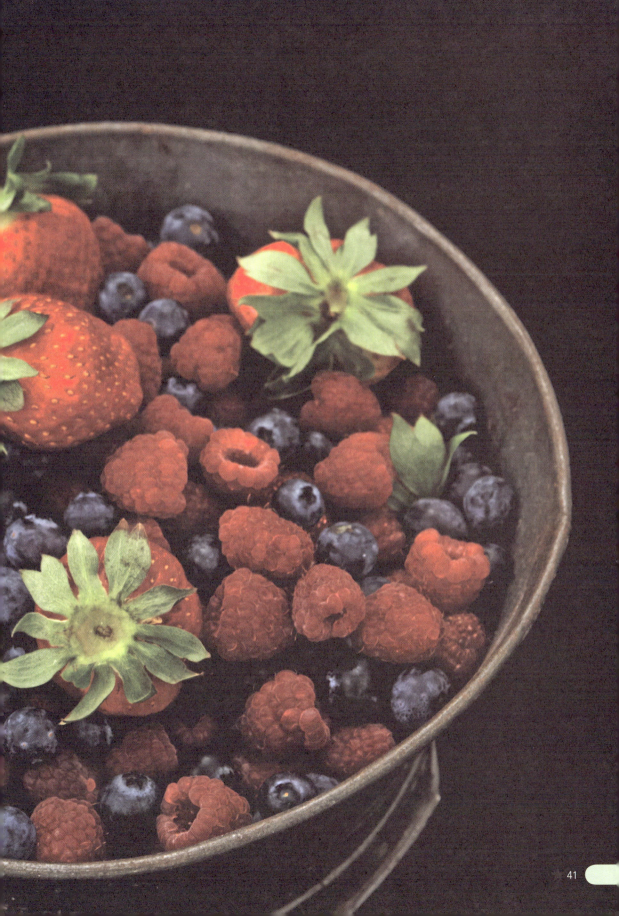

the duration and severity of the infection (Douglas et al, 2004). Our advice is to forget the supplements and tuck into the real thing instead; you'll certainly do no harm this way and just might do much good.

Besides, it's not all about vitamin C. Here are just some of the beneficial nutrients and phytochemicals to be found in these wonderful fruits:

★ Fibre— contributes to its low GI in part due to the good amounts of soluble fibre present as pectin, which slows the absorption of the carbohydrates. The pith also contains insoluble fibre, which acts like a broom sweeping through the intestines, keeping you regular and your gut healthy.

★ Folate—an essential B group vitamin that can prevent neural tube defects in newborns, reduce your risk of heart disease and fight cancer by keeping new cell development healthy.

★ Limonene and coumarin— found in the skin, these are antioxidants which have been shown to stimulate a detoxification enzyme that in turn protects tissues from free radical damage. Don't worry, we're not going to suggest you start eating the skin of your orange, but using the zest in dishes seems a good plan to make sure you reap all the benefits from these fruits.

★ Beta-cryptoxanthin — another of the carotenoid group of antioxidants, found particularly in the orange fruits. Studies are investigating its role in the prevention of colon cancer.

★ Naringin— a flavonoid antioxidant found in grapefruit, and has a role in protecting the lungs from toxins in the air from pollution and cigarette smoke (as does vitamin C).

★ Nobiletin— another flavonoid found in the flesh of oranges and is shown to have anti-inflammatory properties.

★ Tangeretin— yet another flavonoid, this time found in mandarins, is being studied for its potential to reduce tumour growth.

GUAVA

We tend to think of citrus fruit being the best source of vitamin C when in fact guava tops them all. One fruit provides more than double your vitamin C requirements for the day. Guava are also rich in carotenoids, particularly lycopene that is more often associated with tomatoes. There is some evidence to show that a high lycopene intake reduces the risk of cardiovascular disease, certain cancers including prostate cancer, and perhaps also macular degenerative disease. The fibre in guavas is great for your gut and can help to reduce cholesterol levels and the fruit is also a good source of folate, potassium, copper and manganese.

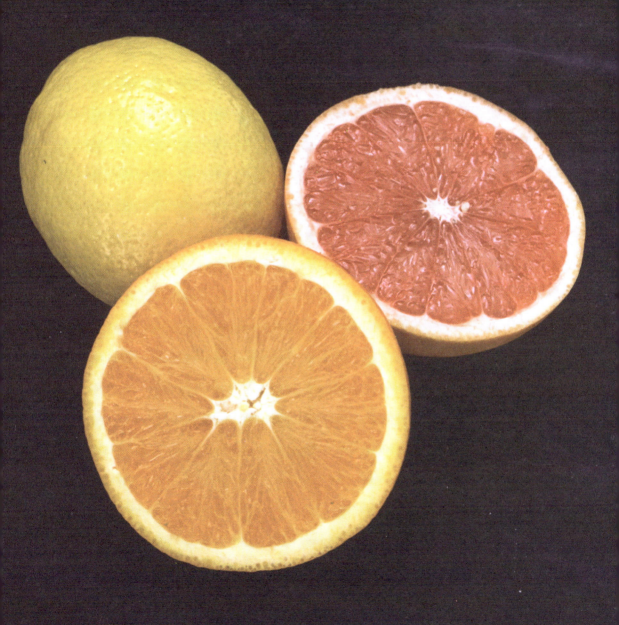

KIWI FRUIT

This strange looking hairy fruit (who on earth first thought it might be nice to eat?!) is one of the richest dietary sources of vitamin C. Just one kiwi fruit provides roughly double the recommended daily intake. Aside from the roles already mentioned, vitamin C also enhances our absorption of non-animal source iron. It is therefore a good idea to slice a kiwi fruit on your muesli or breakfast cereal in the morning, or finish a vegetarian meal with the fruit. A few other goodies to be found below the fuzzy skin are:

- ★ Lutein — one of the carotenoids important for eye health and may also be important in preventing colon cancer.
- ★ Chlorogenic acid — an antioxidant which seems to play a role in preventing tumour growth.
- ★ Fibre — has benefits for the gut and also ensures that the fruit sugars are absorbed slowly, minimising the impact on blood sugar.

MANGO

One of the wonderful things about the start of summer is that mangoes come into season. These delicious tropical fruits are a real treat both in taste and nutrition. They provide several nutrients including vitamin C, vitamin B6 and fibre. Mangoes are also incredibly rich in beta-carotene, much richer than other fruits, and hence the wonderful orange colour. This alone credits the mango as a 5-star performer. Enjoy them sliced on your muesli for breakfast, chopped in a salsa and served with chicken, or try Judy's Avocado, Mango and Pine Nut Salad (page 165).

PAPAYA

The orange colour comes from the presence of carotenoids and there is a good range of the various types in papaya. The fruit is a particularly good source of beta-crytoxanthin, which has been shown in studies to reduce the risk of lung and colon cancers. Other studies have linked this antioxidant to a reduction in the risk of rheumatoid arthritis — a condition also caused in part by free radical damage. Papaya is also rich in vitamin C and the fibre is useful in maintaining a healthy gut and low blood cholesterol. We find the taste of papaya is much improved by squeezing the juice of a lime over the cut fruit.

PASSIONFRUIT

Passionfruit are packed with fibre, providing more than double the amount in the same weight of most other fruits. Aside from benefiting your gut, the presence of soluble fibre can help to reduce blood cholesterol. They are also full of vitamin C and contain good levels of the pro-vitamin A carotenoids. The good levels of potassium can help to lower blood pressure.

PERSIMMONS

Persimmons are not among the most popular Australian fruits but we urge you to be adventurous and try them if you haven't already done so. The rich colour comes from the carotenoids and, in particular, persimmons are rich in beta-crytoxanthin. This carotenoid has been linked in studies to a reduced risk of cancers of the lung and colon, and rheumatoid arthritis. They are also good sources of fibre (twice as much as an apple), potassium, magnesium, manganese and even provide the minerals calcium and iron in useful quantities.

There are two types of the fruit commonly available—the Hachiya persimmon should be eaten when completely ripe and soft, while the Fuyu is smaller and eaten when firm and crisp like an apple. You can eat them raw, mash them up to use in muffins, toss them through a green salad or cook the flesh in a little olive oil, blend and use as a glaze for chicken or meat.

POMEGRANATES

Pomegranates may never have made it to your fruit bowl, probably because many of us don't know what to do with them. That's a shame because they are hard to beat for antioxidant power. If you have never tried one you are in for a treat—both in taste and in nutritional benefit. The word pomegranate actually means 'seeded apple' and this is essentially what it is. The round crimson fruit is packed with clusters of seeds in the same wonderful colour. Pomegranates are rich in vitamin C and fibre and three different types of polyphenols credited with helping in the prevention of heart disease and cancer:

- ★ Tannins—also found in tea and red wine which are responsible for the slightly astringent or bitter taste in these foods. Tannins are better known for their negative effect in binding minerals such as iron, and reducing their absorption. However in the plant, tannins have powerful antimicrobial and antioxidant properties. This has stimulated research into whether these same positive attributes apply when eaten.

- ★ Anthocyanins—a sub-group of the flavonoids and responsible for the purple/red colour of pomegranates; these are powerful antioxidant compounds.

- ★ Ellagic acid—seems to have anti-cancer properties. In laboratory experiments it has been shown to induce cancer-cell death and act as an antioxidant.

Pomegranate juice has hit the shelves in a big way promoting the antioxidant content of the juice. While it does indeed provide these powerful antioxidants, just watch out for the added sugar content. Read the ingredients list to be sure of what else you are getting. As with all fruit juices, they are certainly nutrient-rich but also kilojoule-rich—which won't help your waistline. It is almost always better to eat the whole fruit.

They are not difficult to prepare when you know how. Try this easy method recommended by the Pomegranate Council in California (**www.pomegranates.org**)—they call it 3 step-no mess!

1 Cut off the crown and cut the pomegranate into sections.

2 Place the sections in a bowl of water, then roll out the arils (juice sacs) with your fingers. Discard everything else.

3 Strain out the water then eat the succulent arils whole, seeds and all.

PRUNES

Famous for their ability to promote regularity—prunes are simply dried plums. More energy-dense than the fresh fruit, they are very nutritious—with many of their nutrients surviving the drying process and then concentrated in the prune. Promoting healthy bacterial fermentation and good gut health, their high-fibre content adds bulk to intestinal contents, promoting movement through the gut, and fuel to the bacteria present in the colon. Prunes also have real antioxidant power—containing different phenols helping to protect the fat-soluble areas of the body from free radical damage. Their very low-GI makes them an ideal snack.

ROCKMELON

Rockmelon is wonderfully rich in vitamin C and the orange colour comes from the carotenoids present. It is particularly rich in beta-carotene, containing more than other types of melon. Beta-carotene from foods has been linked to the prevention of cancers and heart disease (taking the antioxidant as a supplement rather alarmingly may have the opposite effect, see page 24 under dark green leafy vegetables). It can also be converted to vitamin A in the body, essential for good vision. Since vitamin A is primarily found in animal fat such as full-fat dairy foods and butter, this can be a good way to ensure you meet vitamin A requirements while reducing your intake of these foods.

Rockmelon is also high in potassium, important in reducing blood pressure, and the soluble fibre pectin, useful in reducing blood cholesterol. Rockmelon may, therefore, help to reduce the risk of heart disease and stroke.

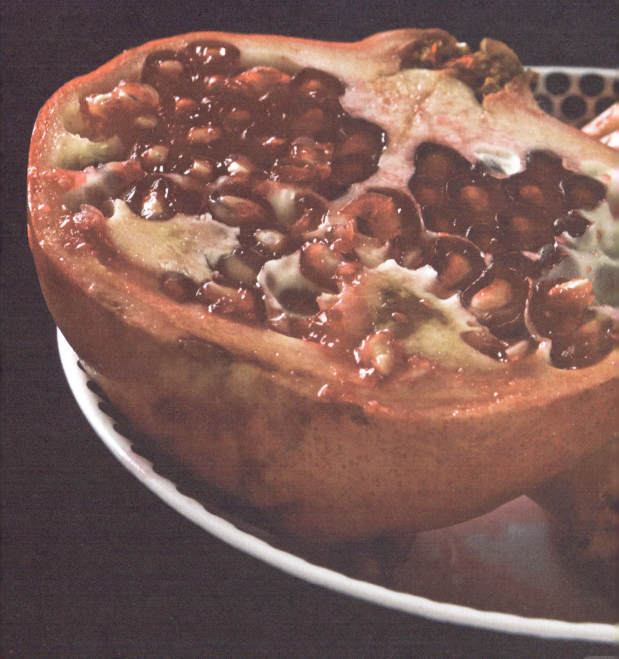

Player Profiles – Fruit

5-STAR PERFORMERS

Fresh Fruit		Nutrient Summary
apricots		Good range of several carotenoids, particularly beta-carotene which, in addition to its antioxidant capacity, can also be used to form vitamin A in the body. Good source of niacin.
avocado		Good source of vitamin K, niacin and thiamin. Higher in energy than other fruits due to high fat content—but the healthy fats that we want (see pages 107–11). The fat content also means that this fruit has excellent levels of fat-soluble vitamin E—itself a powerful antioxidant important in reducing heart disease risk. Great source of fibre.
berries including blueberries, blackberries, cranberries, raspberries and strawberries		All berries are packed with disease-fighting, anti-ageing potential and are hard to beat for antioxidant power coming primarily from the purple/red coloured anthocyanins. High in fibre. All berries are very good sources of vitamin C, vitamin K and manganese. In addition, blackberries contain good levels of vitamin E, folate, magnesium, potassium and copper; raspberries contain magnesium; cranberries have vitamin E; and strawberries have folate and potassium. Wild blueberries, if you can find them, are even more antioxidant-rich. Be careful with cranberries—unfortunately the tart nature of these berries means we have to cook them and add sweetener. This can substantially reduce the nutrients and increase the energy density. However, they do have antimicrobial qualities that can be useful in preventing urinary tract infections. Beware of the juices, which can be very high in added sugar.
Citrus fruit including	grapefruit	Lacks the carotenoids of the pink varieties but remains a 5-star choice providing good total antioxidant power and excellent vitamin C levels.
	kumquat	The essential oils in the peel of citrus fruit contain phytochemicals that have demonstrated anti-cancer effects; for example, limonene increases the levels of liver enzymes involved in detoxifying carcinogens. Since we eat the whole fruit of the kumquat, this lesser consumed citrus fruit may be particularly beneficial. Also a good source of thiamin. They are best stewed with a little natural sweetener added such as apple juice concentrate or honey.
	oranges	Well known for their vitamin C content, oranges also contain a wide range of protective phytochemicals in the flesh, smaller levels in the juice and, as with kumquats, in the peel. Try adding the zest of an orange to a dish or use an orange fruit spread that contains the peel. Also a good source of thiamin.
	pink grapefruit	Packs more nutrition than regular grapefruit thanks to the presence of the carotenoids that impart the pink colour. These include beta-carotene that, in addition to its antioxidant capacity, can be used to form vitamin A in the body, and the powerful antioxidant lycopene also found in tomatoes.
guava		The fruit with the highest vitamin C content by a long shot! The carotenoids present impart the pink colour. These include beta-carotene that, in addition to its antioxidant capacity, can also be used to form vitamin A in the body, and the powerful antioxidant lycopene (also found in tomatoes). Good source of copper and manganese.
kiwi fruit		Only guava contains more vitamin C! Very good source of vitamin K. Good source of vitamin E and copper.
mango		Rich in the carotenoid beta-carotene that, in addition to its antioxidant capacity, can also be used to form vitamin A in the body. Also provides vitamin C, vitamin B6 and plenty of fibre.
papaya		Range of carotenoids present including beta-carotene, lutein and zeaxanthin that are important for eye health, and beta-crytoxanthin, a potent antioxidant linked to lower rates of certain cancers and rheumatoid arthritis. Great for vitamin C and folate and also provides good amounts of fibre and potassium.
passionfruit		Wins the prize for the fruit with the most fibre, providing more than double any other fruit! Very good source of pro-vitamin A compounds such that 100 grams of the fruit provides 25 per cent of daily vitamin A needs. Rich in vitamin C.
persimmons		Particularly rich in the carotenoid beta-cryptoxanthin, which has been shown to reduce the risk of lung and colon cancers, and rheumatoid arthritis. Good levels of vitamin C and excellent for fibre and manganese.
pomegranates		Not so commonly consumed in Australia, which is a shame since this fruit has one of the highest antioxidant levels of all plants! Also provides good levels of vitamin C and fibre.
rockmelon		Particularly rich in beta-carotene that, in addition to its antioxidant capacity, can also be used to form vitamin A in the body. High in the soluble fibre pectin. Good source of vitamin C.

The table below summarises the attributes of each of our fruit players including key nutrients present, the GI where relevant, and any additional information of note.

STAR PERFORMERS

Fresh fruit	Nutrient Summary
apples	Although not the broadest range or spectacularly high levels of individual nutrients, they do contain an array of beneficial phytochemicals. Contain pectin, a soluble fibre that can help to reduce cholesterol as well as helping to lower the GI. Be sure to eat the skin where many of the nutrients and the majority of the antioxidants are found.
bananas	Very good source of several B group vitamins, particularly vitamin B6 and riboflavin. Good source of manganese and potassium. Banned on low-carbohydrate diets due to their higher carb content, but in fact a banana provides only a few grams more carbohydrate than an apple or pear and more vitamin C! At any rate, they have a low to moderate GI making them an ideal snack to tide you over to the next meal.
black grapes	Very good source of vitamin C and vitamin K. The purple colour comes from a group of antioxidants called anthocyanins, which seem to have particular importance in maintaining healthy blood vessels and reducing inflammation.
cherries	The red colour comes from a group of antioxidants called anthocyanins, which seem to have particular importance in maintaining healthy blood vessels and reducing inflammation. Good also for vitamin C and fibre.
green grapes	Very good source of vitamins C and K. Lacks the anthocyanins found in black grapes.
honeydew melon	Not as nutritious as the rockmelon but still a great vitamin C source. Also a good source of vitamin B6.
lychees	Rich in vitamin C and a good source of copper. Avoid those canned in syrup; buy them fresh when you can, or at least canned in unsweetened juice.
nectarines and peaches	Rich in vitamin C and provide fibre. Good source of niacin and potassium and provide beneficial amounts of a range of carotenoids.
pears	Although pears can't boast spectacular levels of any nutrient or phytochemical, they do provide a good fibre and vitamin C boost for very little energy, making them a good choice for a sweet snack.
pineapple	Rich in vitamin C and manganese. Good source of fibre, thiamin, vitamin B6 and copper.
plums	Rich in vitamin C. Good source of vitamin K and fibre. The purple colour comes from a group of antioxidants called anthocyanins, appears to have particular importance in maintaining healthy blood vessels and reducing inflammation.
watermelon	Particularly rich in the powerful antioxidant lycopene (also found in tomatoes) which imparts the pink colour. Ignore the high GI of this fruit; the carbohydrate content per serve is very low making the GI far less important. Fabulous low-energy, nutrient-rich snack.

GOOD PERFORMERS

canned fruit in natural juice	Less nutritious as the skin of the fruit is usually removed and certain nutrients, particularly those that are water-soluble, are lost during the canning process.
rhubarb (stewed with sugar)	We think of rhubarb as a fruit, but it is in fact a vegetable. Raw it packs a powerful nutrition punch, but unfortunately we need to cook it to make it edible and this results in nutrient loss. You also have to add a sweetener and this increases the energy density.

RESERVES

canned fruit in syrup	The syrup substantially increases the energy content and adds a considerable amount of refined sugars. Also less nutritious as the skin of the fruit is usually removed and certain nutrients, particularly those that are water-soluble, are lost during the canning process.

LIABILITIES

none	All fruit has something to offer us and the only liability would be in how they were handled; for example, deep-frying, overcooking and processing.

Vegetables and Fruit

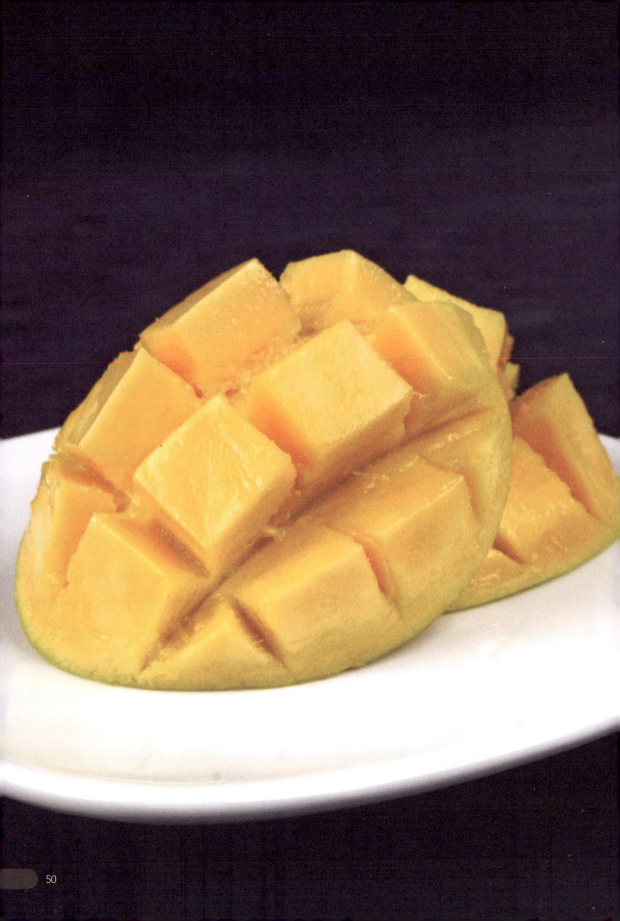

Player Profiles – Dried Fruit

	Dried fruit	Nutrient Summary
5-STAR PERFORMERS	apricot	Fabulous source of antioxidant carotenoids and make a good low-GI snack. Sulphur dioxide is used to prevent browning of the fruit and the growth of micro-organisms. This has been found to be safe at normal levels of intake but, if you are worried, look for organic produce or sundried and get used to the brown colour—the taste is unaffected.
	prunes	Famous for their ability to treat constipation, probably due to the good fibre content and the presence of other compounds which stimulate the gut into movement. The presence of unique phenols and beta-carotene gives prunes an impressive antioxidant power.
GOOD PERFORMERS	apple	Reasonable levels of nutrients and a low GI make these a good snack choice.
	currants	Good for fibre and a plant source of iron.
	dates	Good plant source of iron but their extremely high GI (for Australian-tested dates; other varieties have a lower GI) means they are not such a good choice as a snack. Use in small quantities as part of a meal or as a snack.
	figs	Highest for fibre of all dried fruits—50 grams provides 24 per cent of recommended daily intake. Good non-dairy source of calcium. However the intermediate GI and higher energy density compared to fresh fruit reduces their ranking.
	mango	Unusually for a dried fruit, the vitamin C is preserved. Although no data available for antioxidant power, the combination of vitamin C and carotenoids suggests this would rank well.
	peach	Reasonable levels of nutrients and a low GI make these a good snack choice.
	pear	Reasonable levels of nutrients and a low GI make these a good snack choice.
	raisins	Good levels of nutrients including iron and antioxidant power. Intermediate GI therefore use as part of a meal or mixed with other fruit and/or nuts as a nutritious snack.
	sultanas	Intermediate GI therefore use as part of a meal or mixed with other fruit and/or nuts as a snack.
RESERVES	cranberries	Unfortunately most people find the natural tartness of cranberries unpalatable, therefore sugar is almost always added.
LIABILITIES	none	All dried fruit has something to offer us and the only liability would be in how they were handled; for example, deep-frying, overcooking and processing.

Note: The drying process results in a loss of some nutrients found in fresh fruit and are more energy dense than fresh which is why they fall into the good performing category rather than star. Prunes and apricots provide exceptional other quality benefits and are rated 5-star performers accordingly.

Chapter 3

Carbohydrates

They're in and then they're out. Poor old carbohydrates have taken quite a flogging over recent years as diet after diet hits the shelves blaming these foods for expanding waistlines and almost every chronic disease plaguing the Western world. Yet, health authorities and most dietitians continue to promote a high-carbohydrate diet as the healthy choice. It's little wonder so many people are completely confused about whose advice to follow.

There are elements of truth on both sides of the argument and that is because you cannot simply lump all carbohydrate-rich foods in one basket and say carbs are good or bad. We have to consider the qualities of the individual food before we say if it is a good or bad choice. So what would make a carb a good choice? Take a look at Figure 3.1.

FIGURE 3.1 The best and worst of carbs

The best carbs will	CARBS	The worst carbs will
✓ fill us up and keep us satisfied between meals so that we eat less and don't snack on the wrong things		✗ be rapidly digested and absorbed leading to glucose 'spikes' in the blood after eating which damage blood vessels
✓ deliver glucose slowly and steadily into the blood, keeping our blood glucose on an even keel		✗ lead to a rapid fall in blood glucose an hour or two after eating, stimulating hunger and inducing cravings, especially for sweet foods
✓ be rich in different types of fibre to keep us regular, our bowel healthy and our cholesterol down		✗ stimulate big release of insulin and, if it happens chronically, will increase fat storage, reduce fat burning and is itself a risk factor for heart disease
✓ be nutritionally rich providing an array of vitamins, minerals and phytochemicals such as antioxidants		✗ provide carbohydrate but little else – 'empty kilojoules'
✓ reduce our risk of chronic disease including heart disease, type 2 diabetes and certain cancers		✗ increase our risk of chronic disease including heart disease, type 2 diabetes and certain cancers

Looking at carbs in this way makes it easy to see why there is so much controversy and it also makes it easy to see how we can reap the benefits without the pitfalls. The best-performing choices are obviously those that deliver as many of these attributes as possible. The clear winners are vegetables, fruits, wholegrains, legumes and pulses. These are the least common choices in most Western diets and it is therefore not surprising that carbs have been blamed for many of our ills. Vegetables and fruits are so important, and absolutely essential in any healthy diet, that we have categorised them all on their own. So in this section we will focus on the bigger sources of carbohydrate in our diet—for most that means bread, pasta, rice, breakfast cereal, cakes, biscuits, other grains, legumes and pulses. We'll introduce you to a few you may never have tried, or may never even have heard of, and we'll no doubt disappoint you by relegating a few of your favourites to the 'liabilities' category, but by making better choices more often you have the potential to dramatically change the way you look, feel and perform.

WHY DO WE NEED CARBS?

There are many good reasons to include carbohydrates in your healthy eating menu, including:

★ for optimal **cognitive** performance

★ to perform at our best during **exercise**

★ to maintain a healthy **bowel**

★ carbs are relatively **cheap**, readily available and easy to store.

FOR OPTIMAL COGNITIVE PERFORMANCE

Our brain (and certain other cells in the body including red blood cells) runs almost exclusively on glucose—the carbohydrate that circulates in our blood. While we can make glucose from protein, there is a limit to the rate and capacity to do so. For our bodies to function, blood glucose must not fall below a certain level. If it were to drop dangerously low, we would fall into a coma and, without intervention, could die. That is why our bodies can make glucose from protein; it is a fall-back system to ensure there is a constant glucose supply for the brain. In times of famine, the brain adapts and can run on ketone bodies made from fat, but this is not normal metabolism and certainly not the preferred fuel. Since carbohydrate is clearly an essential fuel in our bodies, it makes sense to bring in fuel in the form it is needed. Research clearly shows that brain function—including memory and concentration—is much improved after eating carbohydrate-containing foods, particularly first thing in the morning. You may have experienced this yourself if you have tried following a low-carbohydrate diet—common complaints are of headaches, lack of concentration and poor memory.

TO PERFORM AT OUR BEST DURING EXERCISE

When we exercise, glucose and fat are used as fuel, but glucose becomes increasingly important as the intensity of the exercise increases. Think of fat as the tortoise—the slow steady burner that can run for a long time but cannot go very fast. Glucose, on the other hand, is the hare—it can produce a lot of energy fast but without refuelling will run out pretty quickly. As we cannot turn protein into glucose quickly enough during exercise, it means we need to have a good store of glucose ready before we start and to adequately fill these glucose stores we need to eat carbohydrate-containing food.

Making exercise a regular part of your life is not an optional extra—it is essential if you want to look, feel and perform at your best. This means that you will need to eat sufficient carbs to support your exercise program. Of course, this also means that the more you exercise the more carbs you need and vice versa; but remember, not exercising and not eating carbs means you miss out on the irreplaceable benefits of both.

TO MAINTAIN A HEALTHY BOWEL

It's interesting that constipation is almost unheard of in native cultures yet is one of the most common complaints in the Western world. Chronic constipation can lead to all sorts of problems including bloating, digestion, abdominal pain, flatulence, haemorrhoids, diverticulitis and bowel cancer. Our sedentary lifestyle plays a huge part in this. An inactive body leads to an inactive gut. A key dietary difference is the amount of fibre we consume.

Fibre is in fact just carbohydrate, but of a type that we cannot break down and absorb in the small intestine. It comes as no surprise therefore to discover the best sources of fibre are also carb-rich foods. If you choose to follow a low-carb diet you inevitably end up with a low-fibre diet and your bowel will suffer as a result.

Fibre acts like a broom through the gut—it absorbs water to swell the gut contents, which in turn stimulates the gut walls to contract and sweep the contents along. Once it reaches the large bowel or colon, it is fermented by the resident bacteria-producing substances that feed the cells of the colon and keep them healthy. Water is reabsorbed here and waste matter eliminated. Modern diets with little fibre contain far more digestible and readily absorbed food. This sounds good but actually means that, by the time the gut contents have reached the colon, there is little left and it moves slowly. More and more water is absorbed making the content drier, more compact and … you get the picture. This means that waste products and potentially carcinogenic compounds hang around longer in the colon where they can do their damage. Gas builds up adding to the problem and you are left feeling bloated, blocked up and sluggish. To avoid this, you need both fibre in your diet and enough water to keep the fibre-rich gut contents fluid.

There are many types of fibre but they are generally classified as insoluble or soluble. Insoluble fibre is mostly found in the outer husk of a grain— the bran. This is removed when grains are polished (for example, in white rice) or processed (for example, to produce white flour). Insoluble fibre is also found in the fibrous parts of vegetables and the skin of legumes, pulses and some fruits. This type of fibre is best for keeping you regular and preventing constipation.

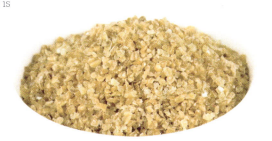

The other major type of fibre is soluble fibre. As the name suggests, this type of fibre is (at least partly) soluble in water and forms a sort of gel in the gut. Soluble fibre is particularly beneficial in two ways. It can 'trap' cholesterol in the gut—both the cholesterol in bile salts secreted by the liver and cholesterol in the foods we eat—and prevent it from being absorbed. This has a small but clinically important effect in lowering blood cholesterol levels. It is for this reason that oats, a grain rich in this type of fibre, are often cited as a good cholesterol-lowering food. Secondly, the gel-like formation slows down the access of digestive enzymes to the carbohydrate present in the gut contents, which in turn slows the absorption of that carbohydrate into the bloodstream. Soluble fibre is therefore intrinsically linked to the GI of the food—foods high in soluble fibre invariably have a low GI. Legumes are a good example of this and one of the reasons they warrant 5-star performer status.

CARBS ARE RELATIVELY CHEAP, READILY AVAILABLE AND EASY TO STORE

From a purely practical point of view, cutting out carbs makes life very difficult, not to mention unsociable. Carbs on the other hand are relatively cheap, you can store them in the pantry making it easier to put together a healthy home-cooked meal without shopping every day, and they are widely available … even your local corner shop will stock bread at the very least. The same cannot be said of fresh protein-rich foods.

Processed high fibre vs naturally high in fibre

Many packaged foods labelled 'high fibre' are not the best choice. Many are simply heavily processed grain foods or have a whole host of other added ingredients, with some bran fibre thrown in to disguise it as a healthy product. Muesli bars are a good example—yes they contain oats and can boast a good amount of fibre, but many also have added hydrogenated fats, syrups and refined sugars which bump up their kilojoule and unhealthy fat content. Many high-fibre breakfast cereals are processed cereals with bran fibre added back in. While they are certainly a better choice than low-fibre cereals, the majority have a high GI since the fibre added is insoluble and does not slow the digestive enzymes.

In fact, there is a major problem with too much of this type of insoluble cereal fibre. It contains compounds called phytates which bind to minerals including iron, zinc and calcium, preventing them from being absorbed by the body. Too much cereal fibre therefore can leave you deficient in one or more of these minerals. The ubiquitous scattering of bran fibre in particular into many of our so-called healthy foods is a double-edged sword—it might be helping our gut, but in those who diligently choose the high-fibre option too often they may be doing more harm than good.

The solution is to choose foods naturally high in fibre rather than too many foods with fibre added. You will then benefit from both the fibre as well as the full array of nutrients that food has to offer. A variety of our top-performing carbs will fit the bill nicely.

The GI—an invaluable tool to choosing quality carbs

Proponents of high-protein/low-carbohydrate diets argue that grains have made us fat. The major flaw in this argument is that we have eaten grains for thousands of years, yet have really only become fat in the last 50. In fact, much of the exponential rise in obesity has been in the last 20 years. Genetic susceptibility undoubtedly plays a part, but cannot explain the full story. We have to question, therefore, what has changed in the last few decades to make us so prone to getting fat?

WHAT DO WE DO TO THE GRAIN?

When man started to eat grain foods, we harvested the grain and would have roughly ground the grain between stones to crack the hard outer shell, added water to the resultant mix and then cooked it in some way. Over time, we learned how to use grain to make bread, cook up porridge or add it to thicken stews. We learned that grains could plump out a meal making the meat in the meal go a lot further while filling everyone up relatively cheaply.

It's the same story today—animal foods tend to be much more expensive while grain foods are cheap and readily available. But we have now learned how to grind the grain, remove the tough outer husk and polish the grain down to just the starch-rich centre. We can then cook the polished grain to give a fluffy white rice, for example, or can grind this starch centre to a fine flour to produce fluffy white breads. Or we take the fine flour and mix it with fat and/or sugar and make biscuits, cakes, crackers, breakfast cereals and so on. You can see that over time, with sophisticated food manufacturing techniques, we have moved further and further away from the grain in its natural state. In fact, all we do is strip the grain of almost all its fibre and micronutrient content, and use only the energy-containing part of the grain—the starchy centre. The real change in the last 50 years has been in what we do to the grains in our diet.

HOW DOES THIS PROCESSING AFFECT THE BODY?

We can measure the effect of this processing on our body and see quite clearly the physiological change. When carbohydrate-containing foods are eaten, the food is digested and broken down in the intestines to release the individual sugars, principally glucose. These are then absorbed into the bloodstream where the glucose is transported to cells all around the body to be used as fuel or stored for later use. How quickly this happens varies depending on the food. This is the basis for the glycaemic index or GI. The GI compares foods, gram for gram of carbohydrate, by directly measuring the rise in blood glucose after eating the food.

In the GI, the response to pure glucose is taken as 100 and all other foods are compared and ranked accordingly. High-GI foods have values of 70 or more (in other words they produce a response equal to or greater than 70 per cent that of pure glucose), moderate-GI foods have values in the range 56 to 69, and low-GI foods have values of 55 or less (in other words they produce a response of 55 per cent or less that of pure glucose).

If we compare directly the GI of grains under increasing levels of processing—wholegrains, cracked grains, wholemeal flour and so on to fine flour—we see a stepped increase in the glycaemic response. Compared to the diets of our ancestors, it is clear that the glycaemic impact today is far greater since we eat far more high-GI foods. In other words, the rises and falls in our blood glucose levels today are far larger than in the past.

Our bodies are just not designed to deal with these rapid and large fluctuations in blood glucose. Glucose levels in the blood need to stay fairly stable and there are systems in place to do just that. When glucose levels rise in the blood after eating carbohydrates, the pancreas releases the hormone insulin. Insulin acts like a key allowing glucose entry into cells around the body. For example, muscle cells take up glucose to use as fuel, or they can store the glucose for later use, the brain needs a constant supply of glucose and the liver also stores some glucose that it can release between meals to prevent blood levels from falling too low. This system works beautifully when there is the right amount of glucose coming in from the gut, the right amount of insulin being released and the right amount of glucose being used up by active muscles. Problems start when the system is overloaded, overworked or malfunctioning.

Overloading happens when you eat a large amount of carbohydrate all at once, and/or carbohydrate that is rapidly absorbed, such as with high-GI foods. A modern breakfast consisting of a large bowl of cornflakes followed by white bread toast will result in overload for most. The system becomes overworked when this happens on a regular basis where modern diets are filled with high-carbohydrate, high-GI foods. The system malfunctions when not enough insulin is produced to do the job, or the insulin produced does not work effectively. This happens in those with insulin resistance and diabetes. In Australia, it is estimated that one in four people have insulin resistance or diabetes (source: Diabetes Australia) and most don't know it. They are a ticking time bomb at increased risk of developing diabetes, heart disease and related conditions. The system also malfunctions when we are too inactive—sedentary lifestyles cause us to lose muscle and this increases our risk of developing insulin resistance.

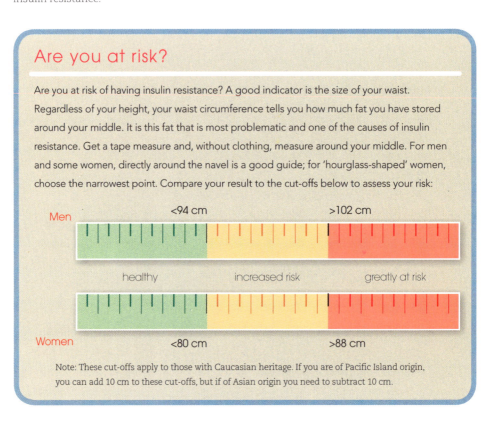

Glucose 'spikes' after eating high-GI meals have been shown to damage blood vessels and cause a low level of inflammation around the body. High levels of insulin are also damaging and hyperinsulinaemia (high insulin in the blood) is a known risk factor for cardiovascular disease. You can control both of these factors by choosing low, rather than high, GI foods at most meals. The occasional high-GI food will do no harm, so long as your overall diet has a low GI. The vast majority of traditional diets around the world do in fact have a low GI, while the majority of high-GI foods are modern processed grain foods that have entered our diet in the last few decades. This is shown in Table 3.1.

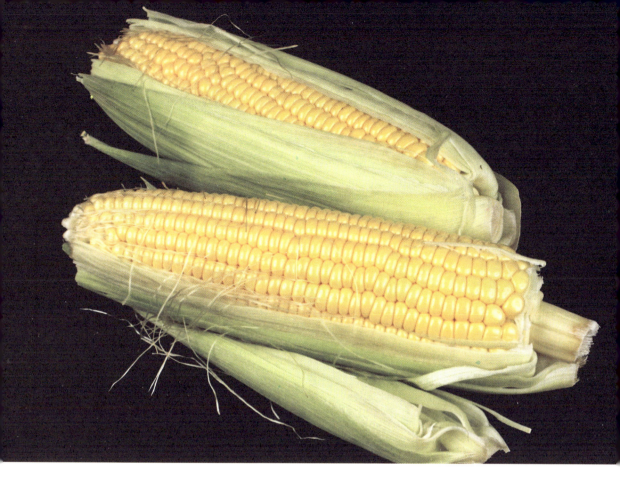

TABLE 3.1 Traditional versus modern GI in foods

Traditional low GI foods	Modern high GI foods
stoneground breads	white bread
sourdough breads	regular wholemeal bread
heavy grainy breads	most polished white rice
porridge oats and muesli	most breakfast cereals
pasta	most cereal snack bars and biscuits
legumes (lentils and beans)	potatoes
most fruit	French fries
barley	scones, pikelets and crumpets
quinoa	bagels
cracked wheat	
buckwheat	
rye	

GI classifications taken from the International Table of Glycaemic Index and Glycaemic Load Values: 2002 (Foster-Powell et al, 2002) and the online database at www.glycemicindex.com.

The GI can sound very complicated and scientific but there is no need to get bogged down in the theory. Neither is there any need to know the GI of every single food you eat. All you need to consider is the GI of the major sources of carbohydrate in your diet—and we have done the planning for you. All of our '5-star performers', and most of our 'star performers', have a low GI. Choose these on most occasions and you will achieve a low-GI diet. It's that simple.

Lessons from the past

One way of determining the optimal human diet is to look back in time. What have we evolved eating and can we compare that to what we are eating now? It is not an easy process to determine what man has eaten hundreds, thousands and millions of years ago, but scientists have good clues and evidence to work with to give us a fair idea. The best evidence points to the fact that man ate an animal-food dominated diet in the pre-agricultural age. This is hunter–gatherer man at his iconic best — the men out hunting wild animals, catching fish and seafood, while the women gathered plant foods such as native vegetables and fruits. Animal foods certainly were the major source of energy but the plant foods provided large quantities of fibre and micronutrients, including antioxidants. Grains would not have been eaten to any large extent at this time, simply because, without modern farming and milling equipment, they would have been too labour intensive.

Then came the agricultural age, so-called because people learned how to farm the land, and grow and harvest crops to support their communities. This happened some 10 000 years ago and from this time cereal grains became an increasingly important part of human diets around the world. When we look at the entire pathway through history of how we have evolved, this is a small step on a very long road. This is the reason why many believe that, genetically, we have not yet evolved to cope with the change from predominately animal-based to predominately cereal-based foods in our diet (Cordain et al, 2005).

If we step forward in time, today we find that almost every community around the world eats approximately the same percentage of their energy intake from protein; 15–18 per cent compared to the estimated 19–35 per cent of our hunter–gatherer ancestors (Cordain et al, 2002). The amount of carbohydrate we eat varies across countries, but grains and foods made from grain are now major dietary players.

At the same time, rates of obesity and chronic diseases are on the increase and, because of this, many believe that we should return to a diet closer to that of our hunter–gatherer ancestors. This is a valid argument and, for some, achieving such a diet may well be advantageous. But there has been a lot of misinterpretation of what such a diet is. The current fad of low-carbohydrate eating takes on various forms but these are not hunter–gatherer diets. There are some key differences:

1. **Fruit usually banned on low-carb diet**

    Fruit is almost always cut out or restricted because it contains sugar, and therefore is bad, yet what can be more natural than eating something that grows from the land, as the 'gatherers' would have done? These same diets will go on to recommend various protein powders and bars, egg replacers and other processed, manufactured food products. How can this possibly be better for us than eating a carbohydrate-containing banana?!

2. **Vegetables severely restricted in type and/or quantity**

    Hunter–gatherers ate large quantities of plant foods, including vegetables. In fact, estimates for their fibre intake are in the range of approximately 90 grams a day, compared to the average of 15 grams a day in Western diets. Diets that restrict vegetables are restricting your fibre and micronutrient intake at the same time.

3. **Differences in meat from domesticated and wild animals**

    Hunter–gatherers ate wild animals, fish and seafood. Today we mostly eat domesticated animals, and even farmed fish and seafood is becoming the norm. There are key nutritional differences between the two, primarily concerning the type of fat present. Meat from animals in the wild tends to be lower in total and saturated fat, and much higher in the fats we know to be good for us, particularly the omega-3 fats. Furthermore, even the type of saturated fat present differs. Saturated fats are classified by their molecular chain length and not all of these fats raise cholesterol levels. It is the shorter chain saturated fats that appear to be responsible. These undesirable fats are the predominant saturated fat in meat from domesticated animals. In contrast, the saturated fat present in meat from animals living in their natural habitat, eating their native diet, is predominately one of the longer chain fats, called stearic acid. This fat does not raise blood cholesterol. This means that a high animal produce diet today is nutritionally different to the high animal produce diet of our hunter–gatherer ancestors.

4 Modern high-meat diets linked to colon cancer

High-meat diets today have been linked to an increased risk of colon cancer (Larsson and Wolk, 2006). The greatest risk comes from eating processed meat products, including burgers and sausages, which would not have been a part of our ancestors' diet, and from eating charred meat. Burning the meat surface produces carcinogens so be particularly careful as to how you cook meat on the barbecue and avoid overcooked, blackened meat. Hunter–gatherer man may have been protected by the simultaneous consumption of high quantities of fibrous plant food. To eat a high-meat diet today, you would be wise to also replicate this aspect of their diet or you risk a wide range of potential gut problems.

Note: The safest way to enjoy your meat is to choose long, slow cooking methods (as in stews, curries and casseroles) and opt for rare or medium–rare when having a steak.

5 What about offal?

If you truly want to eat like a hunter–gatherer, you will also have to broaden your palate past the juicy fillet and include marrow, heart, liver, kidney, brain, intestines and so on. Our ancestors would almost certainly have used the entire animal carcass and been a scavenger of food left over from other animal kills. There are many different nutrients to be found in these different body parts, but are you willing to try it?

6 We drive to the shops to hunt!

The energy needs of hunter–gatherer man were very different. Enormous amounts of energy were expended in hunting and gathering food. It is estimated that today our energy needs are about half that of our far more active ancestors. There are two messages here—firstly that our bodies are designed to be active and need activity to be healthy and, secondly, since most of us will never manage to replicate these extremely high levels of activity, our dietary needs are clearly different.

The argument that genetically we are designed to eat a more animal-based diet is a valid one and we can take some lessons from this. But we can also look at it from a different angle. As man's brain grew so did his capacity for thought and reasoning. We learned how to grow food and thus make it more available and sustainable. Human populations flourished and today the world population is around six and a half thousand million people. We simply could not have grown to this number without grains and other carbohydrate-rich plants to use as food staples around the world, nor could we feed the world population today on a predominately animal-based diet. The fact is that most of the world survives on a carbohydrate-rich diet. Indeed many people around the world, out of choice or food availability, survive and thrive on a completely meat-free diet. One of our survival qualities has been that people can and do survive on a number of different diets depending on the availability of food around. There is not one diet to fit all—you can choose between a number of different healthy diets based on your personal circumstances, health, likes and dislikes, cost and availability of food.

So if you think you would like to follow a diet more like that of our early ancestors, by all means do so but this does not mean a low-carb diet. Cut back, or cut out, grain foods and instead seriously up your intake of vegetables and fruits. Choose a variety of lean cuts of different meats and include fish and seafood several times a week.

WHAT ABOUT SUGAR?

For years we've been told that sugar is bad and complex carbohydrates are good. Contrary to what 'common sense' tells us, foods high in sugar do not have a high GI and those high in complex carbohydrates a low GI. In fact, very often the reverse is true. Sugar is just the name for short chain carbohydrates, while starch is a long chain carbohydrate made up of individual sugars (glucose). Once broken down in the intestine and absorbed into the body, the individual glucose units are all the same whether they came from sugar or starch. The length of the carbohydrate chain doesn't tell us how fast it will hit the bloodstream. An apple is made up of sugars but has a low GI, whereas white bread is starch and has a high GI. The sugar content of these foods tells us nothing about their physiological effect. The key point is that refined and processed carbohydrates, whether they are starch, sugar or a combination of both, are the problem.

Looking at the grams of sugar on the nutrition panel of a packaged food is not helpful as this figure does not distinguish between naturally present sugars in foods, such as in fruit, and added sugar in food. Table sugar is sugar refined from the sugar cane or sugar beet plant. It is really no different to white flour, being the refined carbohydrate portion of the plant. Yet we don't have the same negative associations with flour as we do with sugar. From a glycaemic impact point of view, flour is far worse. Table sugar is made up of two sugars—half glucose and half fructose. The latter does not have an immediate impact on blood glucose as it must first be metabolised by the liver. This is why many foods with added table sugar have low or intermediate GIs. Flour on the other hand is made up of long chains of pure glucose and therefore most foods based on white flour have a high GI.

Nutritionally, eating a lot of table sugar is not a good idea. Table sugar is pure carbohydrate providing energy and no other nutrients; hence you sometimes hear it referred to as 'empty kilojoules'. If we are aiming to maximise our nutrient intake and control our energy intake, taking up 'space' with table sugar is clearly not wise. Sugar does have a place however. It can make some very healthy foods more palatable. You and your children are far more likely to enjoy a bowl of porridge with a sprinkle of brown sugar than without it. And it's far healthier than white bread toast. The bottom line is to look at the overall healthiness of a food rather than its sugar content. Foods with naturally present sugars are not bad for us and, in fact, are usually fabulous choices. A good idea is to use these foods as a sweetener rather than adding table sugar. For example, stir a fruit puree through natural yoghurt for dessert instead of buying yoghurts sweetened with table sugar or artificial sweeteners.

HONEY

Another natural alternative to using sugar is honey. Honey is enjoyed by native cultures all around the world and, from ancient times, honey has been used not just as a sweetener but also as a healing agent. Honey has many qualities that make it a better choice than table

sugar—it has anti-microbial qualities (you can buy honey salves and dressings to aid wound healing), it contains antioxidants and other phytochemicals with health-promoting activities,
it contains small amounts of vitamins and minerals and, if you choose pure floral honeys rather than the supermarket blends, they have a low GI.

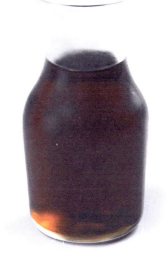

MAPLE SYRUP

Maple syrup is another reasonably good option as it is a natural product. It is made by collecting the sap from the trunks of maple trees and boiling it for hours to reduce it to a syrup. The result is a delicious and low-GI sweetener. Don't confuse the real thing with maple-flavoured syrup—this is less expensive but is also less nutritious, contains undesirable additions and is not low GI.

Conclusions in the great carb debate

★ We have eaten grain foods for several thousands of years without apparent ill effect and, in fact, the ability to survive on crops has sustained an increased world population. From an environmental point of view, we cannot all survive on a meat-dominated diet. The problems have only arisen with the increased consumption of heavily processed grain products, frequently with unhealthy added extras.

★ Wholegrains, legumes and pulses provide us with **key nutrients and fibre** our bodies need.

★ Wholegrains, legumes and pulses are relatively **cheap, readily available and easy to store** making them invaluable as part of a modern healthy diet.

★ The **GI is an invaluable tool** in helping us to make better choices about carbohydrate-rich foods.

★ **Hunter–gatherer man** did not eat grains to any great extent but did have far greater quantities of vegetables and fruits than we do today. These ancestors also ate parts of the animal we may no longer find appetising, and the nutrient profile of today's domesticated animals makes it hard, if not impossible, to truly replicate a hunter–gatherer diet. You can choose not to eat or at least reduce grain foods, but you must seriously up your intake of other plant foods instead.

So, on a thorough study of the evidence, limiting carbohydrates in your diet is not a path to a healthy lifelong diet. Focus on the quality and key nutritional aspects of the whole food instead.

Ranking the Players – Carbohydrates

5-STAR PERFORMERS

Carb Source	
barley—pot and pearl	
beans and lentils (legumes and pulses)	red kidney beans borlotti beans lima beans haricot beans chickpeas cannellini beans butter beans canned bean mix all varieties of lentils mung beans
breads	grainy sourdough pumpernickel traditional stoneground wholegrain
buckwheat	
bulgur	
corn	
freekeh (an ancient green wheat)	
oats and natural muesli	
quinoa	
wholemeal pasta	

GOOD PERFORMERS

Carb Source
chapatti
couscous
doongara rice, basmati rice
millet
mung bean noodles (cellophane)
noodles
pasta
semolina
soba noodles
tortilla
white pita bread
white sourdough breads

STAR PERFORMERS

bran/high-fibre breakfast cereals with low GI
bran/oat muffins with lots of fruit
broad beans
brown rice
mixed grain fruit bread
mountain bread
multigrain English muffins
oatcakes

RESERVES

bagels
dried rice noodles
English muffins, crumpets and pikelets
instant porridge oats
polenta
potatoes
processed low-fibre, low-sugar breakfast cereals
puffed grains
rice crackers, crispbreads and crackers
white bread including baguette, Turkish, Lebanese and focaccia
white rice including jasmine, Calrose and arborio
wholemeal bread

LIABILITIES

commercial cakes, doughnuts and biscuits
commercial fruit muffins
croissants
pappadams
processed low-fibre/high-sugar breakfast cereals and bars

Rolling out the carb players

Each player in the opposite table was assigned a division based on its nutritional profile. The criteria for the selection process were based on their ability to fuel the body for optimal performance. Consideration was given to GI, key nutrients, fibre content, antioxidants/phytochemicals and numerous processing factors.

5-star performer foods for carbs

The 5-star performer foods for carbs give you sustained energy, brain power, concentration, intestinal health and a good night's sleep.

BARLEY

Barley is an ancient grain, being one of the first to be cultivated by man. It has been used as both a staple food and for medicinal purposes since biblical times. Unfortunately, today it has lost popularity as more readily available and processed forms of grains are now the norm and the knowledge of how to prepare grains from their basic form is lost.

> To cook barley as a substitute to rice, soak the wholegrain overnight. Bring 4 cups of slightly salted water to the boil with the grain. Reduce to simmer for approximately 50 minutes or until tender.

Barley, like oats, is rich in soluble fibre and so can be effective in lowering blood cholesterol levels and contributes to good gut health. Barley is a good source of many nutrients including the B group vitamins, especially thiamin and niacin, iron, manganese, phosphorus and potassium. It is available in several forms, most commonly as pearled barley where the bran and outer husk of the grain are removed. Unfortunately, this removes some of the fibre and results in the loss of nutrients. However, it is more palatable in this form and remains highly nutritious. Pot barley (sometimes called Scotch barley) is less refined and contains more of this bran layer, and most nutritious of all is hulled barley where only the outer inedible husk is removed. Pearl barley is widely available but you may have to look for pot or hulled barley in your local health food store. The good news is that all these forms of barley have a low GI and breads made with the cracked grains or intact kernels are also low GI. As with other grains, higher levels of processing increases the GI.

BEANS AND LENTILS (LEGUMES AND PULSES)

Beans and lentils truly are 5-star performers as they provide low-GI carbohydrate, a plant source of protein and iron, are rich in soluble fibre and they even provide a whole host of antioxidants and newly discovered phytochemicals being researched for their ability to protect us from a range of chronic diseases.

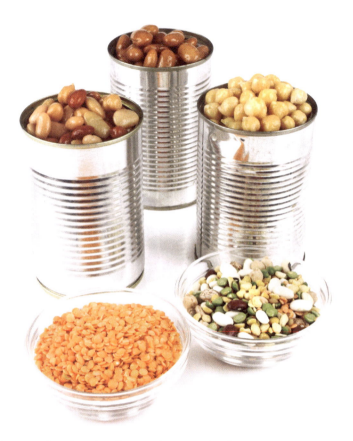

In the West they are often thought of as simply vegetarian fare, and indeed they are invaluable as a protein source in a meat-free diet, but legumes are excellent to replace the more common high-GI carbs in a carnivorous diet.

The biggest hurdle for most people confronted with legumes is what to do with them. They are most often purchased as dried or ready to use in cans. The latter is more convenient as, with the exception of lentils and split peas, legumes require soaking before they are cooked. Cooking them yourself from dried may be more time-consuming but is worthwhile as the beans retain more bite and extra flavour. However, for most purposes, the canned varieties are just as good. Instead of a bowl of fluffy white rice, providing not very much but readily absorbed carbohydrate, opt for a lentil dhal. Or make a chickpea mash to serve with grilled meat in place of mashed potatoes. A bean salsa is delicious with fish instead of boiled potatoes or bread rolls.

Judy swears that adding a strip of the sea vegetable khombu (available from Asian stores or health food shops) can improve the digestibility of the beans and help to prevent flatulence. Sea salt should only be added to the water in the last 5 minutes of cooking (otherwise the skin of the bean will never soften). Once cooked, skim off any froth as this can also cause flatulence and discard the khombu.

Table 3.2 is a guide to cooking legumes and what to do with some of the more well-known legumes (unless stated otherwise, all beans require overnight soaking).

TABLE 3.2 Cooking suggestions for legumes

Legume	Description	Cooking time	Cooking suggestion
Aduki beans	A small red sweet-flavoured bean.	50 minutes – 1 hour	Substitute for meat in casseroles. Popular in Japan.
Black-eyed beans	Mild-flavoured bean, white with a black spot on the end.	1–1½ hours	Delicious with fish.
Black beans	Also called turtle beans.	2 hours	Popular in South America and delicious with spicy Mexican flavours and cool salsas. Delicious in casseroles and soups.
Cannellini beans	White beans of a similar size to kidney beans. Available in cans.	1–1½ hours	Delicious mashed with garlic as a potato substitute. Also good in dips.
Chickpeas (garbanzo)	Round firm-bodied white pea. Popular in Moroccan cooking. Available in cans.	1–1½ hours	Widely used to make hummus. Chickpea flour (besan flour) is excellent for making savoury pancakes.
Green (Puy) lentils (no soaking required)	Puy lentils are native to France and, like champagne, the name is controlled. Australia grows similar varieties, sometimes seen as 'blue' lentils. The lentil is small and green with a delicious nutty taste and holds its shape well.	20 minutes	Delicious in salads, or as a base to fish and lamb dishes.
Kidney beans	A stronger tasting red bean. Available in cans.	1–1½ hours	Used in Mexican cooking. Well known in chilli con carne.
Lentil (red) (no soaking required)	A small orange/red pulse. The archetypal vegetarian food.	15 minutes	Commonly used to make lentil soup. Delicious in dhal and lentil patties.
Lima beans	Also known as butter beans. A large white bean.	1–1½ hours	Serve in soups and winter casseroles.

BREADS

Pumpernickel

Pumpernickel bread is a delicious tasting, heavy dark bread made from wholegrain rye flour and meal. It is low GI, filling and comes in thin slices that are hard to overeat. It's available from most supermarkets, delis and health food stores.

Stoneground

The name comes from the way in which the flour is ground—between pairs of stones rather than the more modern method using steel rollers. This produces a coarser flour with larger fibre particles giving the bread a lower GI. Using the wholegrain also ensures that all the nutrients found in the grain make their way to the bread.

Wholegrain and rye sourdough

The acidic sourdough starter, made by fermenting flour and water over a period of time to use in place of yeast, helps to reduce the GI of this dense and delicious tasting bread. Even white sourdough has a low GI, but only wholegrain and rye sourdough varieties rate as '5-star performers!' being not only low GI but packed with fibre and micronutrients not found in the plain white. Sourdough's popularity is increasing and you can now find many exceptional loaves in delis, health food stores and produce markets all over the country.

Wholegrain bread

Wholegrain bread (where there are lots of visible grain kernels) is both low GI and packed with fibre and micronutrients. Wholemeal is not the same thing—the fibre is so ground down as to make no real difference to the GI. Make sure you can make the distinction between the two when you are buying bread from the supermarket. (Multigrain is really just white flour mixed with a few grains and you cannot be sure of the GI unless it has been tested.) Look for the low GI symbol or buy one that's obviously heavy on grains.

BUCKWHEAT

Buckwheat is described as a grain but is in fact a seed related to sorrel and rhubarb. Although less common in Australia, it has been a staple food for hundreds of years in Asia and Eastern Europe. It is, however, a worthy addition to your diet for several reasons. Unlike most wholegrains, buckwheat is a rich source of all eight essential amino acids. This makes it a particularly good choice for vegetarian meals. It's also good for those with wheat or gluten intolerances being gluten-free and not related to wheat. It is high in fibre, promoting good gut health, and has a low GI. It also tends to lower the GI of bread when added to a flour mix. That may be due, at least in part, to its soluble fibre content which may have further benefits in lowering blood cholesterol levels. Indeed, one Chinese study has shown that consumption of buckwheat was associated with a healthier blood cholesterol profile. Buckwheat is a good source of magnesium, important for healthy blood vessels, and may help to reduce blood pressure, and also contains a range of flavonoid antioxidants that may add to the grain's potential to protect from cardiovascular disease.

Buckwheat can be bought whole and used like rice, roasted (also called kasha), in Japanese noodles (soba) and as flour (the flour is a grey/brown colour). Buckwheat can also be used for a variety of baked products, including pancakes, breads and muffins. People suffering from coeliac disease should avoid buckwheat noodles and pancake mix as they are usually blended with wheat flour. To cook whole buckwheat as an alternative to rice or potatoes, add 3 cups water to 1 cup buckwheat bring to the boil before reducing the heat to a simmer and cooking for 30 minutes or until tender.

BULGUR

Bulgur is popular in Middle Eastern cuisine and is made from whole wheat. The whole kernels are steam-cooked and dried before being cracked into pieces. As a result, it is sometimes known as cracked wheat. Being minimally processed, bulgur has a low GI, making it an excellent replacement for the more common high-GI carbohydrates in Western cuisine such as white rice and potatoes. Bulgur is a highly nutritious grain providing protein, niacin, thiamin, folate and several minerals including iron, zinc and calcium, and as a whole wheat product is high in insoluble fibre important for good gut health. As with other high-fibre grains, bulgur contains lignans—these are phytoestrogens which have come under scientific interest for their involvement in protecting against certain cancers and possibly heart disease.

You can buy bulgur in three different granulations—coarse, medium and fine. You should find it in your local supermarket, sometimes in the ethnic food section or next to the rice varieties, or in health food stores.

> ### How to prepare bulgur
> One great quality of bulgur is that it needs very little cooking. Place 1 cup of bulgur in a dish, cover with 2 cups of boiling water or stock and leave to soak for about 30 minutes, or until all the liquid is absorbed. If necessary, you can drain off any excess liquid.

CORN (whole)

Thank goodness for corn—often the only vegetable our children will eat! Nothing beats a sweet succulent cob of corn and, when you use fresh corn that's sweet and juicy, there's really no need to lather it with butter. Corn was first discovered in Mexico; ears of corns were found in caves dating back as far as 5000 BC and corn remains a staple food throughout Mexico and Central America. Although thought of as a vegetable, corn is in fact a cereal and rich in carbohydrates. We consider it to be a 5-star performer firstly because it is low GI, providing slow-release energy and helping to keep you full between meals. (Mexican corn tortillas are also low GI.) Secondly, when eaten on the cob it is easy to determine your portion size; one cob equals one serving. This makes it hard to overeat and a great alternative to potatoes in a meal. Finally corn is a good source of many nutrients: fibre, vitamin C, phosphorus, manganese and several B group vitamins including thiamin and folate. The yellow colour of corn comes from the carotenoid beta-cryptoxanthin. This antioxidant has been associated with a reduced risk of lung cancer (Mannisto et al, 2004) and rheumatoid arthritis (Cerhan et al, 2003).

When buying corn, check under the husks and avoid cobs with gaps and missing rows. The kernels should be plump not withered and husks fresh, pliable and green. Corn is best during spring and summer—ready for barbecue season. A further advantage is how easy it is to cook; simply remove the husks and all remaining thin fibres and place it in a steamer to cook for 4 minutes until the corn is tender. This helps to preserve the water-soluble nutrients. Rather than smothering the cooked cobs in butter, try drizzling over a little olive or avocado oil. The fat does more than add flavour, it also increases the absorption of many nutrients including the carotenoids. Corn also cans well and is a convenient means of always having some ready to hand for use in sandwiches and salads, thrown into a Bolognese sauce or burger mix, or made into a quick salsa.

FREEKEH

Freekeh (pronounced free-ka) is an ancient Eastern Mediterranean grain. The story goes that in 2300 BC a nation in the Eastern Mediterranean picked the heads of their wheat harvest while still young and green as they needed to store food to see them through an expected siege on their walled city. During the conquest, the store of green wheat caught fire and the outer grains were burned. In an attempt to salvage their food store, they rubbed the heads of the wheat and found this exposed delicious toasted green grains. They called the new style of grain 'freekeh', meaning in their ancient Aramaic language 'the rubbed one'.

The people of the Eastern Mediterranean have eaten freekeh ever since but, until recently, it was not readily available elsewhere. A South Australian company, Greenwheat Freekeh Pty Ltd, has developed unique technology to produce this highly nutritious grain for mass consumption. As a result, 100 per cent Australian grown and produced freekeh is now available—look for it in the health section of your local supermarket or health food store. You can buy it in several forms—cracked grain freekeh, wholegrain freekeh, freekeh flour, freekeh wholemeal flour and freekeh bran.

How to prepare Freekeh

Absorption method

1 cup Greenwheat Freekeh
5 cups cold water

Bring to the boil in a large saucepan, simmer 20–25 minutes (cracked grain) or 45 minutes (wholegrain).

Microwave method

1 cup Greenwheat Freekeh
2 cups boiling water

Place in a deep microwave bowl, cover and cook on high for 10 minutes (cracked grain and wholegrain). Stand for 5 minutes.

Note: 1 cup dry Freekeh yields 3 cups cooked Freekeh.

Nutritionally, freekeh is far superior to many other grains and the more common carbohydrate-rich foods we eat. Freekeh has up to four times the fibre of brown rice, provides more protein than mature wheat and most other grains (similar protein content to pasta made from durum wheat) and is rich in iron, zinc, potassium and calcium. Freekeh is also high in resistance starch—this is starch that cannot be digested and absorbed in the small intestine and therefore reaches the colon where it acts like dietary fibre and contributes to bowel health. This also means the total carbohydrate load of the freekeh meal is reduced, particularly compared to a similar meal using rice or pasta. Not only that, but the CSIRO have been studying freekeh and found both the cracked and wholegrains to be low GI. All in all this makes freekeh hard to beat for those trying to manage their weight, prevent or manage diabetes, reduce the risk of heart disease and promote good bowel health … and that's just about all of us.

OATS (AND NATURAL MUESLI)

In Samuel Johnson's first dictionary of the English language, oats were defined as 'eaten by people in Scotland, but fit only for horses in England'. One Scotsman's retort to this was, 'That's why England has such good horses, and Scotland has such fine men!'

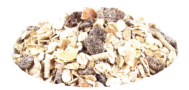

The humble oat is hard to beat when it comes to a complete nutritional package. Not only do oats provide energy-sustaining low-GI carbohydrates, but they are also relatively high in protein. In fact, about 12 per cent of the energy in oats comes from protein making them an especially valuable grain for vegetarians. Fat is high for a grain, providing about 20 per cent of the total energy, but this is almost all healthy unsaturated fat. The fat present also carries fat-soluble vitamin E, a key player in the team of disease-fighting anti-oxidants in the body. In fact, 100 grams of raw oats provides roughly 20 per cent of the recommended daily intake (RDI) of vitamin E for women, and 15 per cent that for men. Oats provide a whole host of other micronutrients including the B group vitamins, potassium, calcium, magnesium, phosphorus, iron, zinc, manganese and the antioxidant mineral selenium.

Along with barley, oats are among the best grain sources of soluble fibre and are renowned for their cholesterol-lowering abilities. Taken together, these attributes make oats a star performer in preventing cardiovascular disease.

Rolled oats are the most commonly available form in Australia. The nutritious outer husk is relatively intact as the grain is lightly steamed and pressed into flat flakes. These are perfect for making your own muesli, soaking overnight for a bircher-style muesli or for a quick-cooking porridge. Don't be tempted to buy instant oats—they may take less time to prepare but are less nutritious with added sugar and flavourings, have a higher GI and won't keep you feeling full for as long. Besides, rolled oats will cook in a few minutes—how much quicker do we need breakfast to be?!

Natural muesli

Oats are the main ingredient in muesli. When you are buying a ready-made muesli from the supermarket or health food store, always check the packaging for added sugar. Sugar listed on the nutritional panel applies to both sugar naturally present in the fruits and added sugar so always check the ingredients. Choose one with no added sugar or oil. Alternatively, make your own using your favourite ingredients or try Judy's recipe on page 147.

Oatmeal is made from ground oats. While less widely available in Australia, it is worth looking out for as it makes a creamier porridge and can also be used to thicken stews and casseroles and to make oatcakes and sweet biscuits. Oatmeal is fine in texture, a creamy colour with golden-speckled particles.

Coarse oats or steel-cut oats are roughly cut groats (the wholegrain). They undergo little processing and consequently are an excellent source of fibre and nutrients. Coarse oats are used to make real Scottish porridge and traditional oatcakes. Traditional porridge involves soaking the grain overnight and cooking in water and salt (a pinch) for up to 45 minutes. As not many people have so much time to spend first thing in the morning, you could save it for the weekend or invest in a slow cooker. Left to cook overnight, you wake to instant porridge for a fraction of the GI. You will struggle to find oatmeal or coarse oats in the local supermarket but you should find them in a good health food store.

Oats will remain fresh stored in an airtight container in a cool pantry for most of the year, but during the hotter summer months they are best stored in the fridge. Use within three months of purchase.

QUINOA

Quinoa (pronounced keen-wa) is a tiny South American grain that has been cultivated for more than 5000 years, and was a staple food of the ancient Incas. It is sometimes referred to as a 'supergrain' given its superior nutrient profile compared to other grains, although it is not really a grain but the seed of a leafy plant. Quinoa is relatively high in protein and, most importantly, the protein is of superior quality because it provides the amino acid lysine, missing in most grains. This makes it an excellent inclusion in a vegetarian diet. Quinoa also has a low GI, and is a good source of iron, potassium and B group vitamins. It is still relatively uncommon in this country but is becoming more widely available as it gains in popularity from health savvy consumers. You will find it in health-food stores and the health section of some supermarkets.

How to prepare quinoa

Quinoa is naturally coated in a bitter compound called saponin. The quinoa you purchase in this country has already had the saponin washed away, but you should give the grains a good rinse under the cold tap to remove any residue. Place the quinoa in a saucepan with one part grain to two parts water. Bring to the boil, reduce to a simmer, cover and cook until the grains become translucent and you can see the spiral germ in each grain. This should take about 15 minutes. As an option, you can toast the quinoa before cooking to give it a nuttier, roasted flavour. Simply heat a non-stick frying pan and toast the grain for about 5 minutes. Cook as above.

WHOLEMEAL PASTA

With four times the iron content and over double the zinc, wholemeal pasta is nutritionally more valuable than white pasta. Both have a low GI compared to other traditionally favoured carbohydrates, but with wholemeal providing over three times the fibre content it's worth adjusting to the taste.

Wholemeal cooks in the same way as white but takes almost twice as long. It has a nuttier flavour so that many people, having made the switch for health reasons, refuse to go back to plain pasta as they prefer the taste.

Look out for pastas (and breads) made from the ancient grains spelt or Kamut®. Both claim to be better tolerated by those sensitive to modern, hybrid wheats developed for their high gluten content. They are nutritionally superior boasting far higher protein and micronutrient contents. They do taste fantastic but the downside is they also cost more.

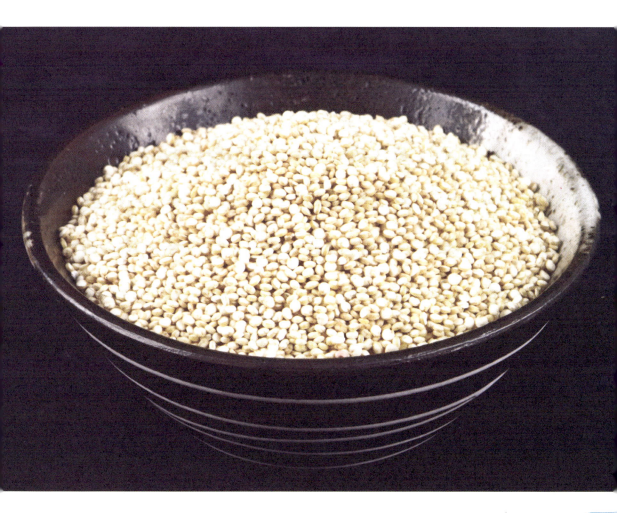

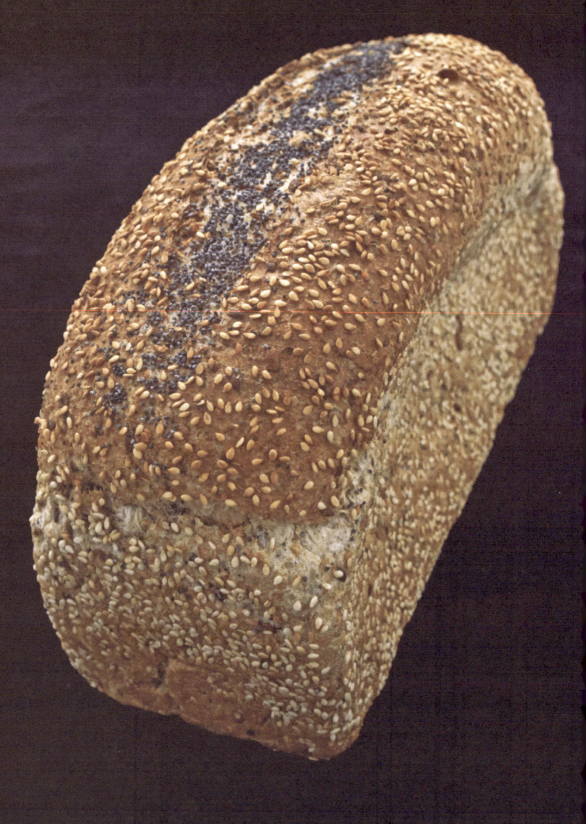

Player Profiles – Carbohydrates

The table below summarises the attributes of each of our carb players including key nutrients present, the GI, processing factors and any additional information of note.

5-STAR PERFORMERS

Carb Source	Nutrient Summary	
barley – pot and pearl	Low GI, provides B group vitamins, good plant source of iron and zinc, and good fibre levels. Can help to reduce blood cholesterol.	
beans and lentils (legumes and pulses)	red kidney beans, borlotti beans, lima beans, haricot beans, chickpeas, cannellini beans, butter beans, canned bean mix, all varieties of lentils, mung beans	Low GI and good source of plant protein, soluble fibre, antioxidants, several vitamins, including folate (borlotti beans a particularly good source) and minerals including iron and zinc. Phytates present do reduce the absorption of these minerals, but this can be improved by consuming a source of vitamin C at the same time.
grainy sourdough	Low GI, high fibre and rich in nutrients. The dense heavy nature makes it very filling and hard to overeat.	
pumpernickel	Made with wholegrain rye flour and meal, low GI, very high fibre and packed with nutrients including B group vitamins and iron.	
traditional stoneground	Low GI due to traditional method of coarse grinding the flour. Look for varieties made with the wholegrain to maximise nutrient intake.	
wholegrain	Low GI, rich in fibre and source of many nutrients including B group vitamins (note that wholegrain is not the same as wholemeal see text on breads, pages 67-8). Look out for breads made from the ancient grains spelt or Kamut®. Both claim to be better tolerated by those sensitive to modern, industrialised wheat and are nutritionally superior boasting far higher protein and micronutrient contents. The downside is they do cost more.	
buckwheat	Provides all essential amino acids making this a great source of protein for vegetarian meals. Rich in fibre, low GI and a good source of magnesium, copper and manganese. Great alternative to rice and ideal for those with wheat or gluten intolerances.	
bulgur	A fibre-rich, low-GI grain and far more nutritious than rice. Great source of manganese, good levels of magnesium and provides significant amounts of several other nutrients.	
corn	Low GI, high in fibre and, particularly served on the cob, corn is an excellent choice in place of potatoes or rice being nutritious and easy to assign an appropriate portion size.	
freekeh (an ancient green wheat)	Higher in protein than regular wheat, low GI, very high in fibre and nutrient-rich. A good non-dairy source of calcium. Available in most major supermarkets in the health food aisle.	
natural muesli	Low GI, added nutrients from dried fruit, nuts and seeds, high in fibre, provides healthy unsaturated fats. Great start to the day.	
oats (traditional)	Low GI and can help to reduce blood cholesterol, probably due to the good levels of soluble fibre present. High in manganese and provides good levels of thiamin, magnesium and phosphorus. Buy the wholegrain traditional variety and not the instant.	
quinoa	A low GI and higher protein grain, packed with nutrients. High in manganese and a good source of copper, iron, magnesium and phosphorus.	
wholemeal pasta	Durum wheat pasta has a low GI and has more protein than many other grain foods. Wholemeal may take some getting used to but is well worth it being nutritionally far superior—rich in fibre, B group vitamins, iron and zinc. Look out for pastas made from the ancient grains spelt or Kamut®. Both claim to be better tolerated by those sensitive to modern, industrialised wheat and are nutritionally superior boasting far higher protein and micronutrient contents. The downside is they do cost more.	

Player Profiles—Carbohydrates (continued)

STAR PERFORMERS

Carb Source	Nutrient Summary
bran/high-fibre breakfast cereals with low GI	The high-fibre content is great for gut health and keeping bowel movements regular—look for one with a low GI (for example, All Bran® varieties) and low added sugar.
bran/oat muffins with lots of fruit	High fibre and lots of nutrients. Good choice for a sweet treat.
broad beans	High GI but not much carbohydrate per serve so this is not so important. Rates highly for antioxidant content and overall good range of nutrients.
brown rice	Nutritionally superior to white rice providing more B group vitamins and a good source of zinc and insoluble fibre, but since most have a high GI it doesn't quite make the 5-star category.
mixed grain fruit bread	Low GI as it replaces some of the flour with dried fruit. This also increases the nutrient content.
mountain bread	Flat bread widely eaten for centuries throughout the world. Available in different grain varieties providing many nutrients. GI varies according to the variety: oat and white both low; rye, barley, rice and organic wheat all moderate; and whole wheat and corn are high. However, since one slice contains about 14 grams of carbohydrate, about half that of a standard sandwich, the overall glycaemic load is less.[1]
multigrain English muffins	Low GI, high in fibre and rich in nutrients from the wholegrain.
oatcakes	Packed with nutritious oats but traditionally made using animal fat. Look for varieties with low saturated fat—those made with olive oil are now available.

GOOD PERFORMERS

Carb Source	Nutrient Summary
chapatti	Traditional Indian flat bread with a low GI. Lower carbohydrate load and less likely to overeat than naan bread.
couscous	Intermediate GI but a little goes a long way making the carbohydrate load per serve relatively small.
doongara rice, basmati rice	Lower GI rice varieties. As with pasta, watch portion size if trying to lose body fat but great carbohydrate source for the very active. Brown rice a better choice for nutrient content.
millet	High GI but good plant source of iron, zinc, B group vitamins and useful for those following a wheat-free diet.
mung bean noodles (cellophane)	Low GI and provides a good plant source of iron and small amounts of B group vitamins.
noodles	Most noodles tested have a low GI and are therefore a good source of slow-release energy. As with pasta, watch portion size and avoid those fried before drying—read the ingredient list.
pasta	Low GI and has approximately double the protein of rice, but be careful with portion size if you are trying to lose body fat. Excellent carb source for the very active. Wholemeal a better choice for nutrient content.
semolina	Semolina is coarsely ground durum wheat before it is used to make pasta and couscous. It is relatively high in protein, has a low GI and provides several nutrients including folate.
soba noodles	Japanese noodles made from buckwheat flour. Although buckwheat is not related to wheat and is gluten-free, these may not be suitable for those with wheat or gluten intolerance as wheat flour is often added to help bind the noodles. Those tested in Japan do however have a low GI, they provide useful amounts of protein and are a good source of manganese.
tortilla	Low GI and although not nutrient-rich, a good way to reduce overall carbohydrate load served as a wrap in place of loaf bread. Unfortunately commercial varieties have added preservatives to lengthen shelf life.
white pita bread	Intermediate GI and less likely to overeat than more fluffy breads.
white sourdough breads	Traditional slow process used and acids present give a low GI. Lower nutrient and fibre count than wholegrain but best white bread option.

[1] The GI values for mountain bread varieties are not listed on the international database but cited from an honours thesis project: Ristevski, S. The Glycemic index of Mountain Bread. Honours Thesis, Department of Agricultural Sciences, La Trobe University results of which are posted on www.mountainbread.com.au.

Carb Source	Nutrient Summary
bagels	Very high GI and high carbohydrate load per serve. Advertised as low-fat but they are energy-dense.
dried rice noodles	High GI and few vitamins and minerals.
English muffins, crumpets and pikelets	Refined carbohydrates with a high GI and easy to overeat. Low-fat but usually served with butter or margarine.
instant porridge oats	The additional processing of the oats increases the GI. Since the traditional varieties take only a few minutes to cook is there really any need for instant?
polenta	GI of 68 so only just avoids being categorised as high GI and usually cooked with plentiful added undesirable fats. However, does provide good levels of certain nutrients.
potatoes	Breeding of potatoes to produce fluffy white produce has led to an extremely high GI. Lower GI varieties are small, waxy potatoes. The nutrients are found mostly in the skin so even less nutrition to be found in mashed and potato products.
processed low-fibre, low-sugar breakfast cereals	Do provide nutrients as these are added but high GI and heavily processed. Really, this is just like eating a processed, nutrient-poor food and taking a vitamin/mineral supplement at the same time.
puffed grains	Puffing grains significantly raises the GI, they are not very filling and neither do they tend to be rich in nutrients.
rice crackers, crispbreads and crackers	Often in a dieter's pantry as being low-fat but highly processed and high GI as a result. Rice crackers may have lower energy than potato chips, but more-ish and, while they may be almost fat-free, they are not energy-free.
white bread including baguette, Turkish, Lebanese and focaccia	Very high GI, made with refined carbohydrate stripped of the majority of the nutrients found in the wholegrain. More-ish and very easy to overeat. Some concerns over residual chemicals from bleaching white flour.
white rice including jasmine, Calrose and arborio	Very high GI and high carbohydrate load per serve, therefore leading to large fluctuations in blood sugar and high insulin demand. Low in nutrients as these are lost in the polishing of the grain. Great for athletes after training but not a good choice for most.
wholemeal bread	Confusing, as this sounds healthy, but not the same as wholegrain. Wholemeal breads often made with mostly white flour with some wholemeal thrown in. More fibre than white but remains as high GI.

RESERVES

Carb Source	Nutrient Summary
commercial cakes, doughnuts and biscuits	Refined carbohydrate as flour and sugar mixed with the unhealthiest types of fat—saturated and hydrogenated vegetable oils. Preservatives, additives and flavourings also usually added.
commercial fruit muffins	So often considered a healthy choice but most are really cakes made from white flour, sugar and a small amount of fruit. To make matters worse, the serve size is usually enormous.
croissants	Combination of refined carbohydrate with lots of the wrong kind of fat. High in saturated fat and can be significant source of trans fat.
pappadams	Fried at high heat and no significant nutrients.
processed low fibre/high sugar breakfast cereals and bars	Often advertise their good vitamin and mineral content, but these are added. It's just the same as eating a bad diet and expecting a multivitamin and mineral pill to fill the gap. Almost all have a high GI and high in added sugars.

LIABILITIES

Note: Soy beans are not included under legumes here as they provide very little carbohydrate. We have included them in the protein group, see page 78.

Carbohydrates ★ 77

Chapter 4

Protein

Protein is found throughout the body—in the hair, skin, nails, teeth, bone, every internal organ and, in fact, virtually every cell. Proteins are also used as chemical messengers, enzymes and nutrient carriers in the blood. It's easy to see why protein is so important in our diet. The question is, how much is optimal for our health and does it matter where we get it from?

The question of how much is not easy to answer. We certainly know how much we roughly need on a daily basis to balance how much we lose; less than 1 gram of protein for every kilogram of body weight. Since the body doesn't have spare stores of protein, as it does for carbohydrate and fat, failing to meet your requirement will mean your body has to pull protein from other parts of the body—usually muscle.

The effects of not getting enough protein are apparent in many parts of the developing world. Protein malnutrition, called kwashiorkor, results in growth failure in children, a loss of muscle mass, decreased immunity, a weakening of the heart and respiratory system and, ultimately, death. In the developed world where a variety of foods are readily available, meeting the physiological requirement for protein is easy. Defining the upper limit for intake is far more difficult.

High-protein diets first appeared in the 1960s but then lost popularity in the wake of the low-fat diet era that followed. The failure of the latter to curb our rising tide of overweight, obesity and chronic disease has led to a striking comeback for high-protein diets. The scientific community were at first slow to respond and most refuted the claims made. However, in the last few years, there has been renewed interest and evidence is emerging to give us a better picture of protein's place in our diet.

There is now convincing evidence to show that a higher amount of protein in the diet can help you to lose weight, improve body composition, help prevent weight re-gain and be beneficial for your heart (Krieger et al, 2006; Halton and Hu, 2004). *What this does **not** mean is that carbs are bad and proteins, whatever the source, are good.* The key aspect seems to be more protein and the diet does not have to be low carbohydrate. Furthermore there are real concerns over long-term effects with at least two recent prospective studies, one from Greece and the other from Sweden, reporting increased mortality, particularly from cardiovascular disease, in those following low-carb/high-protein diets (Trichopoulou, 2007; Lagiou et al, 2007).

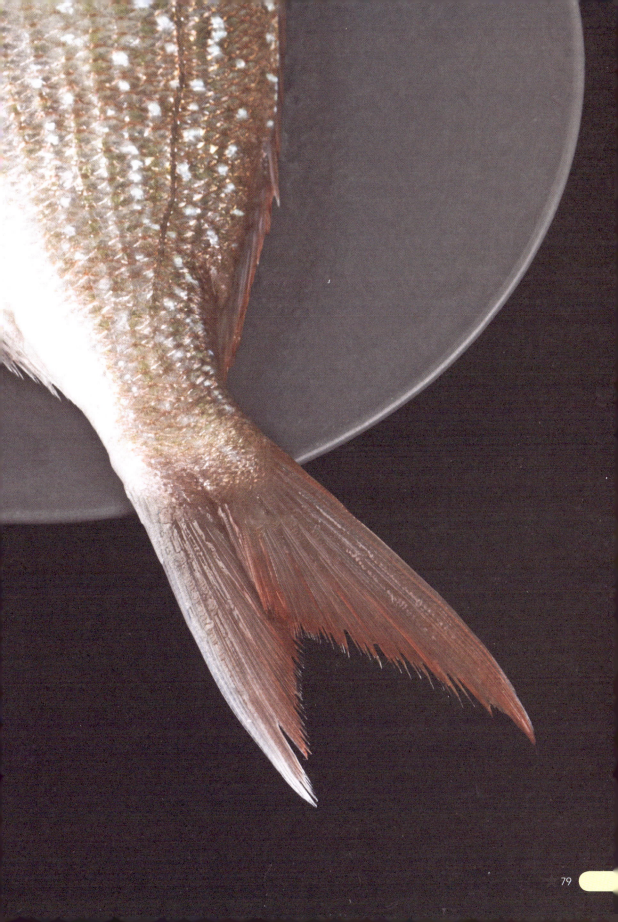

Popular diet books tend to make nutrition all black and white with no shades of grey. They list good and bad foods with rules on how to follow the diet which may seem easier to follow and help to sell books, but there is no evidence to support the safety or efficacy of these diets in the long term. High-protein diets are not all the same; some have high fat levels, some have high fat but low saturated fat, they may be low carbohydrate while others have a more moderate amount of carbohydrate and so on. The same study results from one of these diets does not apply to them all and we can't dismiss the enormous amount of scientific evidence we have concerning fats, fibre, fruits, vegetables, wholegrains and so on. For optimum health, we need to pull all the evidence together to make sensible conclusions on the best diet.

The person who lives mostly on modern high-GI carbohydrates will tend to have large fluctuations in blood glucose (sugar) and a correspondingly high insulin demand on the body. High triglycerides (blood fat), low (good) HDL cholesterol, high insulin and glucose 'spikes' after meals are all a recipe for disaster, increasing the risk of heart disease, type 2 diabetes and related conditions. This does not happen when minimally processed low-GI carbohydrates are chosen and/or *some* carbohydrate is replaced with protein.

Protein can assist in weight control in a number of ways:

- ★ Protein **takes more energy** (more kilojoules) **to digest** and metabolise than carbohydrate or fat.

- ★ Protein is **very satiating** and can help to prevent hunger pangs between meals.

- ★ More protein and less carbohydrate **reduces the glycaemic load** and therefore the subsequent rise in blood glucose. This in turn reduces the amount of insulin required to deal with the incoming 'meal'. With less insulin there is less likely to be a dramatic drop in blood glucose levels 1–2 hours after the meal that can stimulate hunger. And since insulin is a storage hormone—its job is to stimulate the uptake of incoming fat, carbohydrate and protein into cells in muscles, liver and adipose tissue (fat stores)—less insulin around means less stimulus for fat storage and allows for greater fat burning.

But remember, this does not mean you need to cut the carbs completely and neither can you ignore the type of fat. The best evidence supports replacing refined carbohydrates with protein that is low in saturated fat or with low-GI wholegrains or a combination of the two.

Can too much protein be harmful?

Yes. The early explorers of the Americas quickly learnt that if they ate only hunted rabbits with few other foods, they got extremely sick and many died. They called this condition 'rabbit starvation'. Lean meat alone provided them with excessive protein and little carbohydrate or fat. We have a finite ability to metabolise protein and overloading the system results in acid build-up in the blood and, ultimately, death.

To a lesser extreme, eating a lot of protein, particularly animal protein, leads to acidic urine which the kidneys neutralise with calcium. The increase in calcium in the urine is well documented among those following higher protein diets. What is not known is whether this calcium comes from better absorption of calcium from the foods in this diet—and certainly there is some evidence that this occurs when the protein comes from animal foods but not from supplements—or whether calcium is coming from bone. While the jury is still out on the reason, the risk is not worth taking given the debilitating and painful condition of osteoporosis. A point to note is that our ancestors, despite their high-protein diet, appeared to have had extremely strong skeletons. This protection was probably due to their consumption of large quantities of plant foods which buffer the acidity without drawing on calcium stores (Barzel and Massey, 1998). Of course, they were also far more active than we are today and exercise is crucial for healthy strong bones. There are two lessons we can learn here. First, yes we can choose to eat a higher protein diet, but it must be accompanied by plentiful quantities of plant foods. Secondly, that our bodies were built to be active and we absolutely must build exercise into our lives if we want the best health.

A CASE FOR EATING ANIMAL FOODS

We have only to look at our requirement for certain nutrients for pretty compelling evidence of our need for animal foods:

★ The daily requirement for iron is 18 milligrams for women (19–50 years of age) and 8 milligrams for all men and women over the age of 50. It is difficult to meet these requirements from plant foods alone. The best sources of readily absorbable iron are liver, red meat, seafood and other animal foods. By contrast, the iron found in plant foods is poorly absorbed, although helped somewhat by the presence of vitamin C and the body has the ability to increase absorption when iron is needed. Iron is necessary to transport oxygen around the body, in the production of energy to complete physical work and in maintaining a healthy immune system. The symptoms of a low iron intake therefore include fatigue, inability to exercise, an intolerance of the cold and frequent colds, flu and other infections.

★ The daily requirement for zinc is 8 milligrams for women and 14 milligrams for men. While the outer husk of grains does contain some zinc, other plant sources are generally low in this mineral. Animal foods are our best source with seafood and red meat being particularly zinc-rich. Zinc is essential for energy production, in maintaining a healthy immune system, for healthy sperm production in men, for normal growth and development in children, and for healthy teeth, bones and skin. A lack of zinc can lead to skin problems, reproductive defects, immune deficiency, eye problems and osteoporosis.

★ Vitamin B12—only found in animal foods. We are very efficient at recycling this vitamin and so it takes many years of a strict vegan diet to develop a deficiency.

Nevertheless, the fact that a nutrient found only in animal foods is so essential to the functioning of the human body is indicative of the fact that we are meant to eat animal food in some form. Vitamin B12 is essential for the conversion of food into energy, in protein and fat metabolism, for a healthy nervous system, good skin and hair, in the production of DNA and for normal growth and development.

★ Taurine — an amino acid required for successful synthesis of proteins throughout the body. While we can make taurine from other amino acids, there is some evidence that our ability to do this is fairly limited. Taurine is only available in our diet from animal food sources, further weight to the argument.

★ Vitamin A — an important antioxidant and essential for the healthy functioning of the eyes. Yet, this vitamin is not found in any plant food. It is true that certain carotenoids, including beta-carotene, found widely in plant foods, can be converted to vitamin A in the liver. However, there is a limit in our capacity to do so.

★ The types of fat available to us from plant and animal sources are different. Only animal foods have the **longer chain fats** essential for the normal functioning of all cells in the body. While we can make these longer chain fats from the shorter plant fats, we are less efficient at doing so. This applies to the omega-3 fats we know to be important in brain development and function — those present in plants such as linseeds are shorter chain than those found in oily fish and do not have quite the same effect. (They are still beneficial and a good option for those who can't or won't eat fish and/or seafood.)

This is not to say that you cannot follow a vegetarian diet. You can indeed do so, provided you take great care in your food choices to provide all the nutrients you need. The stricter you are with the foods you avoid, the harder this becomes. If you choose to follow a vegan diet, you would do well to use animal-free supplements to ensure you meet all nutrient requirements. What this evidence does suggest is that, genetically, humans have evolved to rely on animal produce for key essential nutrients. If you choose to be vegetarian or vegan, do so for personal, moral or religious reasons, but not with the belief that it will necessarily be healthier. Equally, it is clearly important for meat-eaters to be discerning about the protein foods they eat regularly and they must also be sure to include sufficient plant foods for balance.

Type of protein

The building blocks of protein are the amino acids of which around 20 are important in human metabolism. Every protein in the body is made from particular combinations of the amino acids. Some of these we can synthesise from other amino acids, while some must be obtained from our diet. The latter are called the essential amino acids. The protein in our food contains various quantities of amino acids. Animal foods, including dairy foods, contain all of the essential amino acids and are known as complete proteins. Plant foods, in contrast, almost always lack or are low in one or more of the essential amino acids. This is not a problem provided a variety of different plant foods are consumed across the day. For example, grains are low in the amino acid lysine, but if you eat your bread along with hummus or lentil spread you will obtain your lysine from this source. These are sometimes called 'complementary proteins'. The exception is soy protein. This does contain all of the essential amino acids and, for this reason, is often used in protein powders and is an alternative infant formula for babies intolerant to cows' milk. If you are vegetarian, soy beans and soy produce such as tofu and tempeh are smart additions to your diet.

We must also pay attention to the other nutrients that come along with the protein in foods. Many animal-sourced protein-rich foods are also fat-rich foods, and much of this fat is saturated.

Only a few of the currently popular high-protein diets recognise this and make specific recommendations about the type of fat. The vast majority have pushed the low-carbohydrate ideal without consideration as to the quality of the foods that remain. This is exactly the same mistake as was made early on with the low-fat era of dietary recommendations. We must stop these ridiculous, one-eyed diets that blame one macronutrient for all our ailments. In choosing foods we should be more concerned with quality and nutritional value of the food, rather than obsessing over the macronutrient content. The bottom line is that we need quality carbohydrates, quality fats and quality proteins to look, feel and perform at our best.

Ranking the Players – Proteins

Rolling out the protein players

Each player was assigned a division based on its nutritional profile. The criteria for the selection process were based on their ability to maintain, support and strengthen the body for optimal performance. Consideration was given to the quality of the protein, key nutrients, fats present and processing factors.

5-STAR PERFORMERS	Protein
	chicken and turkey breast—skin removed
	eggs—free range or organic
	fish—especially oily
	game meats, for example kangaroo and venison
	lean pork
	lean red meat
	liver
	low-fat milk and natural yoghurt
	seafood (excluding prawns, squid and fish roe)

STAR PERFORMERS	Protein
	cheeses naturally lower in fat, for example, ricotta, cottage
	legumes and pulses
	natural yoghurt (full fat)
	prawns, squid and fish roe
	smoked fish
	soy

GOOD PERFORMERS	
	organic low-fat sausages and burger patties
	textured vegetable protein (TVP)
	veal

RESERVES	
	chicken thigh, leg or wing
	duck and goose
	fatty cuts of red meat
	full-fat cheese
	(low and full-fat) flavoured yoghurts
	full-fat milk
	reduced-fat and manufactured low-fat cheese

LIABILITIES	
	commercial burgers and sausages
	cured meats, for example prosciutto and bacon
	diet yoghurts
	salami

The 5-star performers for protein

CHICKEN AND TURKEY

Chicken has become such a popular meat that chicken producers have of course searched for ways to produce greater quantities of meat for a cheaper price. There have been numerous scare stories in the media. In particular, there is a widespread belief that chickens are fed hormones to promote rapid growth and that this is causing horrendous health effects in both children and adults. This is just not true. Hormones have been banned from chicken production since the 1960s. *Regardless of which type of chicken you choose to purchase, be assured that (at least in Australia) it does not contain growth-promoting hormones.* Nevertheless, while it could be argued there are few differences from a nutritional standpoint between birds raised free range or in an intensive farming practice, undeniably the former taste infinitely better and, from a humane standpoint, the birds have lived a happier life. So just what is the difference between conventional, free range and organic?

Conventional commercially produced chicken

Birds are raised in large sheds (they are not kept in cages) and do not have access to outdoor areas. The area or range per bird is considerably smaller than free range or organic.

While no hormones are given to the birds, antibiotics are used although under strict industry codes. The Australian Chicken Meat Federation (ACMF) states that antibiotics are used to perform two functions; to treat bacterial infections in unwell birds, and to prevent infections or diseases in well birds. They state that antibiotics are not used to promote or enhance bird growth. There are also strict withholding periods to ensure that there is no residue left in the meat at the time of processing. Chicken meat is regularly tested to ensure that this is the case. Concerns have been voiced over whether the use of antibiotics in chicken farming increases the numbers of antibiotic-resistant strains of bacteria, which may threaten human health. However, provided you prepare and cook chicken products correctly, all bacteria, resistant or otherwise, are killed making any cross-contamination extremely unlikely. In addition, the antibiotics used are not the same as those used in humans, although these are permitted when there is no alternative for specific treatment.

Finally, the feed used varies. For commercially reared birds, this is predominantly grain-based where pesticides, insecticides and artificial fertilisers are likely to have been used, and may also contain genetically modified crops.

Free range chicken

The major difference with free range chickens is in their living conditions. Birds are allowed access to an outdoor run during the day and the area or range per bird is considerably larger than for conventional commercially reared birds. The other major difference is that, in buying free range produce, you can be assured that antibiotics have not been used at any stage in the birds' life. Antibiotics can be given to treat disease, but the meat from these birds can no longer be sold as free range. The feeding practices are similar to conventional commercially reared birds. The certifying body for free range chicken meat in Australia is Free Range Egg and Poultry Australia Ltd (FREPA). All certified meat must comply with their standards. You can view these and get more information at www.frepa.com.au.

Organic chicken

Organic chicken comes from birds with similar living conditions to free range; that is, they have access to an outdoor run during daylight hours and have far more space than conventional commercially reared birds. The key differences here are, firstly, that the feed used must be 95 per cent organically certified. This means no genetically modified crops and no pesticide and insecticide use. Secondly, the birds cannot be treated with antibiotics and neither are they routinely vaccinated. Producers must comply with the National Standard for Organic and Bio-Dynamic Produce and bear a certification logo from an approved organisation.

In deciding which type of chicken meat you buy, price will undoubtedly be a factor with conventional chickens being the cheapest and organic produce costing up to three times as much. The reason is quite simply that the organic farming method costs more—more space per bird and more expensive feed for starters. We wholeheartedly support the organic philosophy and believe that this is the best option where possible, taking all factors including animal welfare into account—not to mention taste. From a nutritional point of view there may be small differences. Allowing birds to roam outside feeding on grass as nature intended, can increase the omega-3 and vitamin E content of the meat and eggs. Nevertheless, put the additional benefits of organic produce versus perceived dangers of conventional into perspective. There is little point in spending the extra on organic chicken for your family if you then also load the shopping trolley with packets of biscuits, bottles of soft drink and stop on the way home for a fast-food burger!

EGGS

Eggs were once in, then they were out and now no one really knows where they stand. Are eggs healthy or not? Well, the confusion has come about because of the many sides to the humble egg. On one hand, the egg comes pretty close to being the perfect food providing many of our required nutrients. The white is almost entirely protein and contains all of the essential amino acids we need, while the yolk contains numerous vitamins and minerals (so please don't throw it away!). On the other hand, they are high in cholesterol and the yolk is a considerable source of fat providing 65 per cent of the total energy of the whole egg.

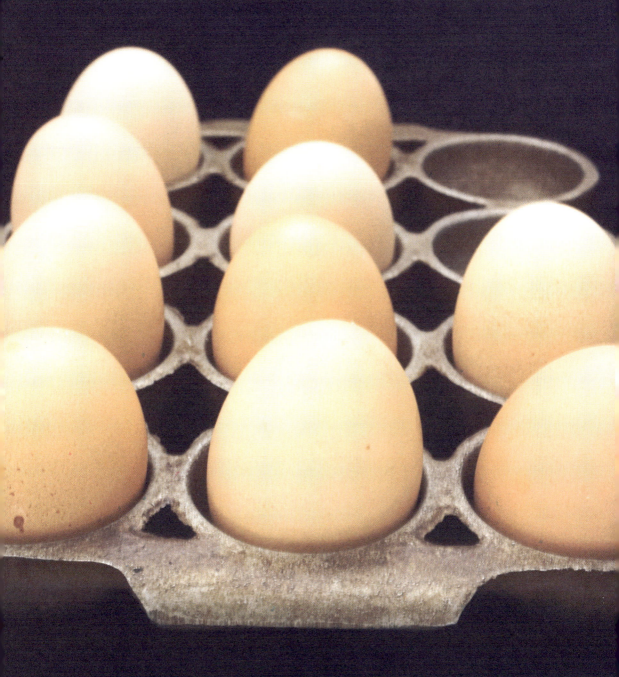

When it was first realised that blood cholesterol levels were related to heart disease it seemed a logical jump to assume that cholesterol in foods would have a major impact on blood cholesterol levels. This led to the advice to eat less cholesterol and eggs hit the 'bad' foods list. Add to this the obsession with eating low-fat foods and eggs had certainly lost favour. However, scientific research later showed that the major dietary influence on blood cholesterol is saturated fat with dietary cholesterol having far less impact. The reason for this is that cholesterol in the blood comes from both diet and cholesterol produced in the liver — if you eat less cholesterol your liver will produce more and vice versa. Saturated fat on the other hand affects how much cholesterol the liver produces. Current dietary advice to maintain healthy cholesterol levels therefore focuses on reducing saturated fat and replacing it with healthier unsaturated fats.

> ### What's in an egg?
>
> **1 medium sized egg (48 grams) provides:**
> 300 kilojoules (70 calories)
> 5.3 grams fat, of which 1.4 grams is saturated fat
> 206 milligrams cholesterol
> 0.1 gram carbohydrate
> 6.2 grams protein

Eggs contain around 5 grams of fat each, but less than half of this comes from saturated fat. The type of egg you buy further influences the type of fats present. Free range eggs may have a healthier fat profile than cage eggs. One study compared the nutrient profile of eggs from a US supermarket (from battery hens fed a commercial feed) with those from a Greek village (free range hens fed a traditional grain diet) and they found a phenomenal difference in the type of fats present. The Greek eggs contained less saturated fat and far more of the healthy fats, especially the omega-3 fats (Simopoulos and Salem, 1989). These are known to reduce your risk of heart attack, are important in maintaining healthy blood and are essential for brain development and function. The feed given to the hens is clearly a crucial factor here and certainly you can now purchase cage eggs high in omega-3s. However, since we also know that exercise affects the fat levels in meat this may also make a difference to the fats found in eggs — free range hens are clearly more active than caged. This subject is hotly debated with egg producers arguing an egg is an egg. We say free range hens must be happier and this is reason enough to buy their eggs. If we also get better nutrition so much the better.

So, not only are eggs not 'bad' but they can make a significant healthy contribution to your diet. If you already have high blood cholesterol you are probably best to limit yourself to around 4 per week but, otherwise, if you like to have eggs for breakfast then go ahead and enjoy. But be careful with the added extras — butter in scrambled eggs or cheese in an omelette can add a lot of the wrong kind of fat. Otherwise go for poached or boiled eggs and add your choice of wilted spinach, grilled tomatoes, mushrooms and wholegrain or sourdough bread. Delicious!

Egg definitions

Cage eggs

These eggs account for most eggs sold in Australia. They come from hens kept in battery style cages with little room or freedom for movement.

Vegetarian eggs

Most consumers see 'vegetarian' and assume therefore that this is a healthier egg. In fact, in order for eggs to be vegetarian, the hens must be on a completely animal produce free diet and this means they cannot be allowed to roam free range where they naturally forage for insects and worms outdoors. These eggs are therefore usually from cage-kept hens simply fed a vegetarian diet.

Barn laid eggs

These are from hens that are housed in a large shed rather than cages. They have enough room to walk around and flap their wings, but do not have the same space as free range birds.

Omega-3 eggs

These are from hens fed a diet high in omega-3 fats and vitamin E to boost the content of these essential nutrients in the eggs. These may be either free range or cage-kept hens—read the label to be sure. Those labelled 'naturally richer in omega-3s' are usually from hens allowed to roam free range and consume a more natural diet including grass.

Free range eggs

These are from hens with access to an outdoor run during daylight hours. The hens therefore have more space than cage-kept hens. Behind organic eggs, free range eggs enriched with omega-3s are the next best choice.

Organic eggs

These are eggs from hens fed certified organic feed; that is, feed grown without the use of pesticides, insecticides and artificial fertilisers. The hens cannot be fed antibiotics and conditions must comply with strict humane practice codes. These eggs tend to be naturally richer in many nutrients including omega-3 fats and vitamin E due to the high quality of feed used. They will, however, be more expensive as a result.

FISH

All fish is 5-star performing for protein as it is low in saturated fats and a good source of many nutrients including niacin and other B group vitamins required for energy metabolism. Fish also provides iodine, an essential component of thyroid hormones; iron for healthy red blood cells and oxygen transport; zinc, essential for many metabolic processes and a strong immune system; and small quantities of folate, essential in the production of DNA and new cells in the body.

Oily fish gets a special mention as these are the best sources of the omega-3 fats we now know to be more than just good for us, but essential for looking, feeling and performing our best. Oily fish include salmon, trout, mackerel, sardines, tuna, herring and kingfish. Omega-3 fats help to prevent blood clots and thus reduce your risk of heart attack and stroke. They also have an anti-inflammatory effect and research has shown benefit to those with rheumatoid arthritis. Upping the intake of fish omega-3s may also help in other inflammatory-related or auto-immune conditions including asthma, pulmonary disease, multiple sclerosis, psoriasis and inflammatory bowel disease. For more information on omega-3 fats see page 109.

Mercury in fish

One concern with increasing fish consumption is the mercury content. Increasing levels of mercury in our waters has occurred through industrial pollution and this mercury then builds up in the flesh of certain fish. All fish contain some trace of mercury but it is the larger fish at the top of the food chain, or those with a longer life span, which accumulate higher levels. The greatest risk is to the unborn child, infants and young children. In babies, high exposure to mercury seems to, albeit subtly, affect attention, memory and learning. For this reason, women planning a pregnancy, those who are pregnant and young children should take care with which fish to consume on a regular basis. (Very little mercury is transferred in breast milk.) In adults it takes a lot more mercury to cause any symptoms—tingling in the lips, fingers and toes is usually the first sign—but this is extremely unlikely to occur as a result of eating fish within health guidelines.

Fortunately, Food Standards Australia New Zealand (FSANZ) have found that most fish caught and sold in Australia are low in mercury. Fish found to have the highest levels were billfish (swordfish, broadbill and marlin) and shark, followed by orange roughy (sometimes called sea perch) and catfish. FSANZ make specific recommendations for limiting these fish, particularly for those pregnant or planning pregnancy and young children, but stress that fears over mercury content of fish should not outweigh the health benefits of consuming more fish.

(For more information visit the FSANZ website **www.foodstandards.gov.au**.)

The bottom line is this, steer clear of the fish listed above if you are worried, or stick within the FSANZ recommendations, but choose from any other fish at least two times a week.

Did you know?

One hundred grams of cooked octopus has more than double the iron content of 100 grams of cooked lean beef, but has 30 per cent fewer kilojoules (or calories), only a trace of saturated fat (compared to approximately 3.5 grams in lean beef) while both provide similar amounts of protein.

A dozen oysters is not only an elegant (and hopefully romantic) entrée to choose, but provides almost 10 times the daily recommended intake for zinc, half that for iron and niacin, about a third for magnesium and almost all the phosphorus an adult needs. All this for only 550 kilojoules (130 calories) and 4 grams of fat.

A dozen mussels provide your total daily requirement for iron, a third that for zinc, more than a third of your magnesium and a tenth of your vitamin A needs, while providing only 540 kilojoules (130 calories), almost no saturated fat and less than 3 grams total fat.

Half a medium-sized lobster provides only 630 kilojoules (150 calories), just over 1 gram of fat, and almost no saturated fat while supplying 32 grams of protein. Compare this to a medium-sized chicken breast (skin removed) with 1100 kilojoules (260 calories), 11 grams of fat of which 3 grams is saturated fat and only a few more grams of protein. The lobster also provides seven times the iron and more than double the zinc of the chicken breast.

GAME MEATS

Game meats include kangaroo, emu, ostrich, venison, hare, rabbit, goat, buffalo (bison), quail, pigeon, partridge, grouse, pheasant and guinea fowl. You have probably never tasted or even seen some of these meats and not all are readily available in Australia. However, if you travel to the US, Europe or many other parts of the world, many of these become more common. Here in Australia, kangaroo is our own unique game meat and is becoming increasingly popular as health-conscious consumers realise how fabulously healthy, and tasty, it is. You should also be able to find fairly readily several of the other game meats and it is worth experimenting with these new tastes and flavours in your journey to better health.

So, why are game meats so fabulous? These are the closest meats we can find today to match those eaten by our hunter–gatherer ancestors. Although most are now farmed to some degree, this is far less intensive than the more popular domesticated animals, and many continue to be 'hunted' in the wild. This means antibiotics and hormones are not used in their rearing, they eat their native diet and exercise far more than their domesticated relatives. As a result, game meat is generally incredibly lean, almost without exception low in saturated fat, a good source of omega-3 fats, high in protein and with none of the concerns surrounding the intensive rearing of farm animals.

The downside is that, being harder to find, less popular and less intensively reared, they can also be more expensive (although not necessarily, so shop around). The exception here in Australia is kangaroo. You can now buy it in most supermarkets and butchers and it is great value, being far cheaper than most other quality meats.

Whichever meat you choose, we always advocate choosing quality over quantity. Use the money you save from cutting down on commercial packaged foods to spend on fresh quality foods such as this. So, don't compare the price of a kangaroo fillet to a bag of processed meat sausages—in terms of 'bang for your bite' the kangaroo wins hands down and your body will thank you for it.

> **Note:** Due to the low fat content, kangaroo and goat meat can lose moisture and toughen quickly if exposed to high dry cooking. The meat should be marinated before roasting or cooked in wet dishes.

TABLE 4.1 Comparing meats

Per 100 grams cooked meat	Energy in kilojoules (calories)	Protein (grams)	Fat (grams)	Saturated fat (grams)	Iron (milligrams)	Zinc (milligrams)
venison	664 (158)	32.9	2.8	1.2	4.8	3.3
kangaroo	612 (146)	32.0	1.8	0.6	4.2	3.6
goat*	600 (143)	27.1	3.0	0.9	3.7	5.3
rabbit	712 (170)	29.3	5.7	2.2	1.3	2.1
beef rump	765 (183)	28.5	7.6	3.4	3.4	4.5
pork fillet	655 (156)	30.9	3.5	1.4	1.5	2.5
trim lamb	749 (179)	30.5	6.2	2.7	5.4	4.8
veal	596 (142)	31.6	1.6	0.5	1.8	3.7
quail	826 (197)	27.7	9.6	2.5	1.8	1.3
emu	516 (123)	25.7	2.2	0.7	2.9	1.0
ostrich*	464 (111)	32.2	1.2	1.0	4.9	4.9
chicken breast (no skin)	660 (157)	28.1	5.0	2.3	0.8	1.4
turkey breast (no skin)	648 (155)	29.4	4.0	0.9	0.6	1.9
duck (no skin)	765 (182)	24.3	9.5	2.8	2.6	2.9
liver, lamb	972 (232)	30.6	10.7	3.1	8.1	5.5
liver, chicken	666 (159)	25.7	5.5	1.8	7.3	4.0

Note: Analysed using Foodworks Professional (Xyris software 2005) using Australian and New Zealand data
* No Australian data therefore figures from USDA database.

All of these meats make a valuable contribution to a healthy diet. They are all relatively low in saturated fat, some extremely so, they provide similar amounts of good quality complete protein and all are a source of the essential minerals iron and zinc. That said, some meats stand out as truly exceptional choices. Venison, kangaroo, goat, emu and ostrich really stand out, providing very low fat and saturated fat, but exceptionally good levels of iron and zinc, for relatively low kilojoules. Venison and kangaroo are the most widely available in Australia and New Zealand. Ostrich is growing in popularity in both the US and Europe as consumers become aware of its phenomenally healthy profile. If you get the chance to try it, do take the opportunity.

If you are feeling tired and suspect you may be low in iron, without doubt your best choice is liver. If you also want to keep the kilojoules and saturated fat down, chicken liver is better than lamb while still providing phenomenal levels of iron—more than double that of a beef rump steak. Unfortunately, many of us are not big fans of liver, while liver products such as pâté tend to have added undesirable fats such as butter and cream. A word of warning too for pregnant women who need an iron boost, liver contains a massive amount of vitamin A—almost four and a half thousand times the recommended daily adult intake in lamb liver and almost 900 times in chicken liver! Such enormous amounts can be damaging to the developing fetus and for this reason all pregnant women should avoid liver and liver products. For everyone else, if you like it, an occasional liver meal will give you an incredible nutrient boost.

Of the more common, widely available meats, you can see that all of the lean cuts listed make pretty good choices. Beef rump or fillet and trim lamb cuts are the best for iron and zinc but beware that, if you choose fattier cuts, the saturated fat content can jump four-fold. Veal is very low in saturated fat and an excellent source of zinc. Chicken and turkey breast are great protein sources with very little saturated fat, particularly turkey, but these have far lower levels of iron and zinc. Duck tends to be much fattier, but if you remove the skin the saturated fat content is on a par with trim cuts of red meat and you get more iron and zinc than the other poultry options.

LEAN PORK

Apparently pork is the most widely eaten meat in the world, although in the West beef tends to be more popular. There are, of course, religious restrictions for some that will negate its place here. Note that we don't include pork products such as ham and bacon in the 5-star performing category, but fresh lean pork cuts such as fillet. This ensures you get top quality protein with very little total or saturated fat. Pork is also incredibly rich in the B vitamin thiamin, necessary to convert our food into energy for use by the body, essential for normal growth and development and to maintain healthy functioning of the heart, nervous and digestive systems.

LEAN RED MEAT

While overt nutrient deficiencies are relatively uncommon in the developed world, one we still see widely is iron deficiency. This is in part due to our relatively high requirements for iron and the fact that so many of us simply don't eat enough iron-rich foods. Children and both pre-menopausal and pregnant women are particularly at risk given their higher requirements for the mineral. You also have increased requirements if you regularly give blood, have any sort of intestinal bleed (for example, an ulcer) or are recovering from an accident where you lost a substantial amount of blood. Zinc is another mineral we have relatively high requirements for, but is often low in diets, particularly when no meat is eaten.

Red meats, as we can see in Table 4.1, are without doubt the best sources of both of these minerals and this is the major reason why we rate them in the 5-star performers category. If you choose lean cuts and trim away any visible fat, you get all the protein, iron and zinc with only small amounts of saturated fat. It is well worth finding a good butcher in your area who stocks grass-fed (may be listed as pasture-fed) meat rather than grain-fed. The latter are fattened up on grain meal to encourage marbling of the meat—that is, fatty streaks throughout the meat which makes it impossible to remove. Chefs may well choose this type of meat as the fat helps to keep the meat moist and undoubtedly adds flavour but, if you want to keep your saturated fat intake down, go for the grass-fed lean option. You just have to be more careful with cooking methods and you will find this type of meat to be delicious while incredibly nutritious.

LIVER

Not to everyone's taste, including ours we must confess! However, there is no denying that liver is packed with essential nutrients including all the amino acids we need. In particular, liver is the best animal source of iron, containing 7–8 milligrams per 100 grams, roughly double that of most red meats. It is also rich in zinc, necessary for a strong immune system and often lacking in modern diets, and a very good source of vitamin C, riboflavin, niacin, vitamin B6, pantothenic acid, folate, vitamin B12, phosphorus, copper and selenium. Liver is extremely rich in vitamin A

This is good for most of us as it is necessary for good vision, among other things. However, since high levels of vitamin A can cause deformities during fetal development, pregnant women should avoid liver and liver products including pâté. It can be quite fatty depending on the source (lamb's liver has more than double the fat of chicken liver) and be careful with liver products such as pâté, which have significant added fat, much of it saturated. It is also high in cholesterol. This is not a problem for most as your saturated fat intake is far more likely to affect your blood cholesterol levels than how much dietary cholesterol you eat, but those with high cholesterol should limit their intake. Despite these flaws, we feel it has to be a 5-star performer given the rich nutrient mix it has to offer. Furthermore, if you believe in trying to follow a diet as close to our ancestors as possible, it's fairly certain liver would have been a prized food.

LOW-FAT MILK AND NATURAL YOGHURT

Milk is considered such an important food in Western countries that, along with the various dairy products made from it, it merits a food group all to itself. Yet, the vast majority of the rest of the world does not drink milk beyond infanthood. This paradox has led to furious debates on the healthfulness of milk with fervent believers on both sides.

On a positive note, milk packs a whole lot of nutrition into one easy-to-consume and inexpensive package. The nutrients present include calcium, vitamin D, vitamin A, vitamin B12, niacin, riboflavin, potassium, phosphorus, good quality protein providing all the essential amino acids we need, and low GI carbohydrates. The fat in whole milk is high in saturated fats, but that's easy to avoid by choosing a low-fat milk from the vast range available.

Of all the health claims, the one that probably comes to mind is that drinking milk is good for your bones. The risk of osteoporosis is increased in those with a low calcium intake, and it's hard to beat dairy products for easily absorbable calcium. Add to this the fact that vitamin D and phosphorus are also crucial for maintaining strong bones and milk does indeed look pretty good. You can, of course, get your calcium elsewhere and in parts of Asia where they consume no dairy products and have far smaller daily intakes of calcium, they also have less osteoporosis. However, there are many other differences that may account for this including higher activity levels, genetic factors and their daily exposure to sunlight (needed to stimulate vitamin D production in the skin). Nevertheless, if you don't like, can't or don't want to consume dairy products you can obtain your calcium from dark green leafy vegetables, dried beans, fish (where you also consume the bones, for example, sardines, anchovies or whitebait) and seafood.

Milk is also good for our teeth. After consuming milk (or other dairy foods), oral acidity is reduced and saliva flow is stimulated. This reduces both tooth erosion and plaque formation. The presence of key minerals such as calcium in the mouth also binds to the tooth enamel. Together, these factors mean stronger teeth and fewer dental caries.

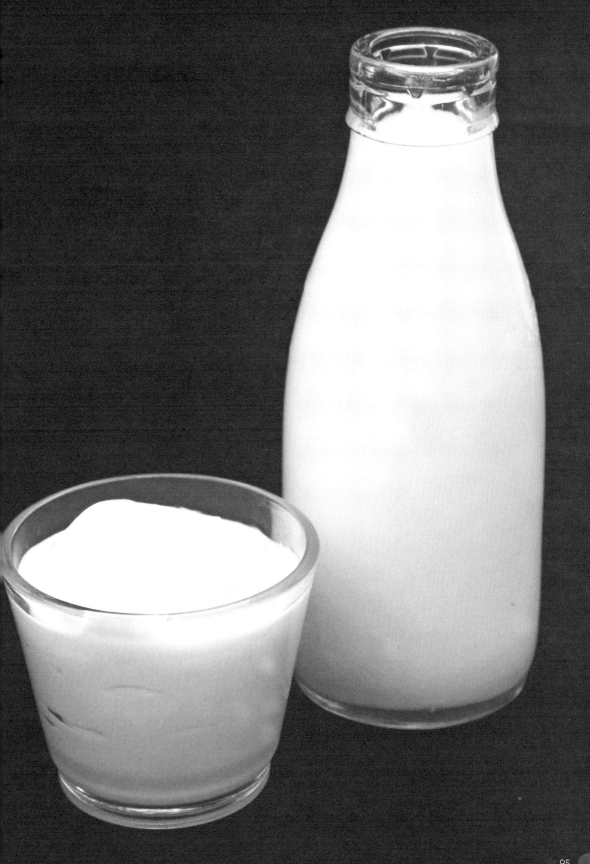

If you think that milk is fattening, you may have to think again. A number of epidemiological studies have shown that those with the highest intakes of calcium from dairy foods have lower weight for their height. In fact, dairy may help you to lose weight. Several controlled clinical trials have shown that three serves of dairy a day assists in weight and fat loss when consumed as part of an energy-restricted diet. Dairy foods may also help to reduce weight gain, especially that seemingly inevitable middle-age spread. While discussions of the potential mechanisms involved have centred around calcium, when supplements are given in place of dairy foods the same results are not found (for a review of the evidence, see Zemel, 2005). While not all studies concur with these findings, it does suggest that there is something about dairy foods that goes beyond the calcium they provide.

Milk and dairy proteins have also been shown to lower blood pressure and large-scale population studies have shown that those with the greatest milk and dairy food intake have the lowest blood pressure (Jauhianen and Korpela, 2007). While two studies in the US have reported that dairy foods may protect against the development of type 2 diabetes and its precursor, insulin resistance syndrome (Lui et al, 2006; Choi et al, 2005).

All sounds good for milk so far, so why the controversy? Milk is more often than not among the first foods to go in popular detox diets and many alternative health practitioners in particular advise against consuming dairy. Many claim that milk increases mucus and nasal congestion, but scientific blinded trials refute that this is the case. It may simply be that the creamy feel of milk in the mouth gives this impression. Nevertheless, anecdotally many people report improvements in their condition when they avoid dairy foods so it is certainly worth a go if this affects you. Similarly, science research has failed to find any link between dairy foods and asthma. Be careful therefore not to unnecessarily restrict your diet or that of your child's before taking known risk factors into account.

You may have seen a new type of milk on your supermarket shelves called A2 milk and wondered what it is all about. Milk contains many different proteins which can be divided into two general types; whey and casein. The A1 and A2 refer to different types of casein present in milk. Standard milk contains a mixture of these two caseins, whereas A2 milk contains almost entirely A2. According to the research, this is the type of milk produced by all cows thousands of years ago, before widespread domestication of cattle. A1 appeared as the result of a random mutation in European cattle and subsequent breeding has resulted in most of our milk today containing a mix of A1 and A2. Why might this be important? Epidemiological evidence has shown an association between A1 consumption and type 1 diabetes (not the more common type 2) and heart disease. No association was found for A2 consumption. A1 intake has also been linked to autism and schizophrenia. Subsequent animal studies provide supporting evidence for these observations, but we need more evidence to be sure of the effects in humans. Anecdotally there are reports of better tolerance of A2 milk in those intolerant to regular milk. However, be wary—if you are allergic to regular milk you are almost certainly allergic to A2. There is currently intense and heated debate over A2 milk, not least because should the hypothesis prove to be correct the dairy industry will be forced to make major changes. At the time of print Food Standards Australia New Zealand state 'both A1 and A2 milk are safe and nutritious for most people'. It's a case of watch this space on this one. For more information read Professor Keith Woodford's book *The Devil in the Milk* or go to www.a2corporation.com and if you are convinced sufficiently to pay a little extra for A2 milk, it is available in most major supermarkets.

There is also some concern that a high dairy food intake may increase the risk of two cancers:

1. Some studies, but not all, have found that high levels of galactose, a sugar released when lactose in milk is digested, may be damaging to the ovaries and raise the risk of ovarian cancer. However, reassuringly, a recent pooled analysis of studies showed no associations between any dairy food and ovarian cancer and although there was a slight increase in risk with the equivalent of three or more servings of milk a day, this was not statistically significant (Genkinger et al, 2006).

2. A Harvard study found that a high calcium intake (not necessarily from dairy) may be a potential risk factor for prostate cancer (Giovannucci et al, 2007).

These findings are by no means conclusive but they do merit taking a cautious approach. In fact, they confirm what can be said of many foods and nutrients, that some is good but more is not always better and may even be harmful.

There are two solid reasons to avoid milk: if you have an allergy or intolerance to milk or if you just don't like it. Allergies to milk (usually to the proteins present) are relatively uncommon and are usually found in children who, more often than not, grow out of their allergy. Far more common is milk intolerance and this is usually to the type of carbohydrate found in milk called lactose. In order to digest lactose, we need the enzyme lactase. Without it lactose passes undigested into the colon where it is fermented by the resident bacteria. The symptoms manifest as abdominal pain, diarrhoea and excessive gas after eating lactose-containing food. Infants almost always produce lactase but, with the exception of Caucasians, most races cease to produce it beyond childhood. This gives a physiological explanation as to why milk remains an important food for Caucasians, originating from Europe where milk and dairy products are widely eaten, while most other cultures of the world do not drink milk. If you are lactose intolerant you may find you can tolerate yoghurts containing live bacteria as these break down some of the lactose for you.

The bottom line is, as most of the world does not drink milk we can clearly live without it. But, if you like milk and milk products and have no problems digesting them, then what fabulous nutrient and protein-rich foods to choose. We have, therefore, ranked low-fat milk and natural yoghurt as 5-star performing protein choices. These are unadulterated with sweeteners or flavours, can help suppress your appetite between meals making them great for snacks, provide the most readily absorbable form of calcium, provide complete protein and so are particularly great for non-meat eaters and they are all low GI.

SEAFOOD

Similar to fish, most seafood provides good levels of omega-3 fats as well as being high in protein and low in fat, particularly saturated fat. All seafood is an excellent source of various micronutrients similar to fish, but is an even richer source of the minerals iron and zinc. Oysters and mussels score particularly well on this front being rich in both minerals. In fact, oysters are the richest food source of zinc, containing approximately 10 milligrams per oyster, while mussels have more than double the iron content of red meat. This makes them an excellent choice for those who wish to avoid red meat, while still meeting requirements for these essential minerals. Other nutrients found in seafood include potassium, needed to maintain healthy blood pressure; phosphorus, for strong bones and teeth; and magnesium, needed for proper nerve and muscle function and heart health. For those who don't eat dairy products, oysters, prawns and scallops become a valuable source of calcium.

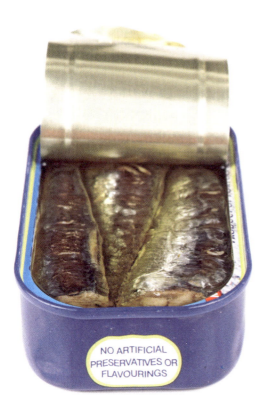

Many people avoid seafood in the belief that it is high in cholesterol but, in fact, this is only true for prawns, squid (calamari) and fish roe. We also now know a lot more about how dietary factors affect our blood cholesterol levels and cholesterol in our diet is far less important than the total amount of saturated fat. Soluble fibre in the diet also helps to prevent dietary cholesterol from being absorbed and so by eating these foods in the context of a plant-rich, high-fibre diet, they are far less likely to have a detrimental effect. Furthermore, given that these foods provide omega-3 fats and many other nutrients, they need not be avoided on the basis of their cholesterol level. Nevertheless if you have been diagnosed with high cholesterol, it is prudent to limit your intake of prawns, squid or fish roe to no more than once a week, but you can happily choose from the many other types of seafood on a more regular basis. For this reason, these three types of seafood don't quite make it to our 5-star performer category, but remain a good choice.

Soy

Soy is a health food, right? So why is it not in our 5-star performer category? Beneficial effects of soy have been reported in relation to heart disease, breast cancer, prostate cancer, menopausal symptoms, thyroid function, bone health and even cognitive function. Yet, conversely, media reports and numerous websites claim exactly the opposite. Frightening headlines touting 'the truth about soy' allege soy is toxic to humans and causes numerous detrimental health outcomes including reproductive problems, an increased risk of breast and prostate cancers, decreased immune function, gut problems, and in children early menarche and feminisation of boys. It's enough to turn you off your soy latté for life. But who do we believe?

Soy is a legume that is fairly unique in the plant kingdom in that it provides all of the essential amino acids (the building blocks of protein) that humans need. In contrast, almost all other plant foods are missing or low in one or more of these amino acids, meaning that vegetarians must consume a variety of plant foods to meet their protein requirements. For this reason, soy beans, tofu, tempeh, soy drink and other soy foods have long been a mainstay of vegetarian and vegan diets. But, on the whole, soy foods have not played a major role in the typical Western diet. In contrast, soy is regularly consumed by many Asians at all stages of life from weaning to old age. This difference in levels of soy consumption is what got the ball rolling in soy research. Scientists found that levels of heart disease and many cancers, including breast cancer, were far lower in these soy-eating Asian countries, compared to levels in the West. Numerous studies followed to try to identify what it was about soy that might be protective.

Research has centred on two aspects of soy—soy protein and compounds found in soy called isoflavones. Isoflavones are phytoestrogens (meaning 'plant oestrogen') and are similar in structure to the hormone oestrogen. These phytoestrogens can act in two ways:

1. They can act like oestrogen. This may be beneficial during menopause, for example, when natural oestrogen levels are dropping. Theoretically, consuming sufficient phytoestrogen-rich soy at this time can reduce menopausal symptoms.

2. They can block the action of oestrogen. This is potentially beneficial in, for example, breast tissue where oestrogen stimulates growth of both normal and cancerous cells. At least one of the isoflavones in soy, called genistein, has been shown in animal studies to inhibit the development of breast cancer.

Additionally, isoflavones have been shown to be powerful antioxidants and may in this way contribute to protection against diseases including cancer and heart disease.

Soy and heart disease

In 1995, a report was published in the prestigious *New England Journal of Medicine* that concluded (on the basis of 38 controlled clinical trials) that soy protein significantly reduced blood cholesterol levels, particularly LDL ('bad') cholesterol, and triglycerides (another blood fat linked to an increased risk of heart disease) (Anderson et al, 1995). On the back of this report, the US Food and Drug Administration now allows food manufacturers to claim on the labels of low-fat foods containing at least 6.25 grams of soy protein that soy can help reduce the risk of heart disease. Many other countries, including the UK, have followed suit but as yet Food Standards Australia New Zealand (FSANZ) have not approved such a claim here and it is unlikely that they will. A more recent review of the evidence published in the journal *Circulation*, suggests that this claim is rather premature (Sacks et al, 2006). It concludes that soy protein has only a very small effect on LDL-cholesterol, reducing it by a meagre 3 per cent or so, while having no effect on triglycerides or 'good' cholesterol. Furthermore, the studies showing a beneficial reduction in cholesterol used large quantities

Soy (continued)

of soy—approximately 50 grams a day. In reality, this equates to drinking about seven cups of soy drink or eating close to 600 grams of tofu every day! You would have to be pretty dedicated to keep up this level of intake. Nevertheless, the authors did recognise that consuming soy foods in place of animal foods (high in saturated fat and cholesterol) should benefit heart and overall health since soy foods are low in saturated fat, a source of healthy unsaturated fats, and rich in fibre and other nutrients. All this research is really telling us is that having soy drink instead of milk and the odd tofu burger is not enough to bring down your cholesterol levels. But, choose the tofu burger over a regular burger, and replace the fattier cuts of meat in your diet with tofu or tempeh, and your heart will be thankful.

Soy and cancer

Some of the early studies comparing cancer rates across countries showed a benefit of soy consumption, and many soy and health food companies leapt on the results. However, the picture is far from clear and a few worrying reports have emerged suggesting that concentrated soy supplements in fact stimulated cancer growth in subjects with existing breast cancer. Of course, this so often happens in nutrition research—scientists think they have isolated the important component of a food and try giving it as a supplement and lo and behold the effects are not the same. Try as we might, a good diet just cannot be packaged in a pill.

The Cancer Council has issued a position statement to help clarify the research information we have on soy and give the best advice possible to consumers. They state that:

- a high consumption of soy foods may lower the risk of breast and prostate cancer, but only by a little
- there is no association between soy foods and the risk of any other cancers
- while they may have a protective effect, there is also some evidence that phytoestrogens might stimulate the growth of existing hormone-dependent cancers (that is, the risk is if you already have hormone-dependent breast cancer and consume a lot of soy).

They therefore recommend that soy foods be included in a healthy high plant food diet, but that soy or isoflavone (the isolated phytoestrogens) supplements should *not* be used to prevent cancer or be used by cancer survivors. Furthermore, if you have or have had breast cancer, they recommend you do not consume a large amount of soy food. For more information visit The Cancer Council website www.cancercouncil.com.au.

Soy and the menopause

Many women have sworn that eating more soy foods during the menopausal years has helped to reduce symptoms such as hot flushes and mood swings. However, the vast majority of studies have failed to confirm these anecdotal findings. Yet it is interesting to note that the reported incidence of hot flushes differs across countries with varying soy intakes. For example, while 70–80 per cent of European women report hot flushes, only 18 per cent and 14 per cent do so in China and Singapore respectively. These differences are perhaps due to the way in which soy is consumed—not as supplements but as key foods in an overall healthy diet.

Soy and reproductive health

Reports of girls starting menarche at an increasingly young age and the feminisation of our boys and men are among the more horrific of the claims made against soy. The basis for this is legitimate enough—that if infants are fed soy formula and young children consume soy in an increasing number of foods they are exposed to the effect of an oestrogen-like substance for a far longer period of time. Certainly infants in Asia are rarely given soy formula, but they are fed many soy foods from the age of weaning. These children have no ill effects on their reproductive systems and there seems little concern from soy foods. With respect to soy infant formula, a major study published in 2001 in the *Journal of the American Medical Association*, followed more than 800 men and women fed soy formula as infants into adult life (Strom et al, 2001). They found no significant differences between this group and those fed a cow's milk formula, including any effects on the reproductive system. That said, there are those who seem to believe soy formula is healthier and there is simply no basis for this.

The bottom line is that breastfeeding infants has indisputable advantages to bottle feeding, but modified cow's milk formulas are a safe and effective alternative. Soy-based formulas were developed for use in infants allergic or intolerant to cow's milk and therefore only consider using them if advised to do so by your doctor or health professional.

The soy bottom line

While there seems little evidence to support the alarmist claims of the anti-soy network, neither is there compelling evidence that soy is quite the health food some have cracked it up to be. The traditional Asian diet, rich in soy foods, has been shown to be a healthy diet that undoubtedly plays a role in their low rates of several chronic diseases including heart disease, obesity and certain cancers. What they don't do is take concentrated soy or isoflavone supplements, nor do they consume a plethora of processed, packaged foods marketed as healthy just because it is made from soy, alongside a diet too high in saturated fat, processed foods and so on typical of many Westerners. Traditional soy foods such as tofu, soy drinks made from whole soy beans, tempeh and whole soy beans are healthy additions to your diet, particularly if they replace processed and fatty meats. But there appears to be nothing to be gained, and potentially much to lose, from trying to take the easy route and package soy in a pill.

Player Profiles – Proteins

5-STAR PERFORMERS

Protein Source	Nutrient Summary
chicken and turkey breast—skin removed	Great source of protein that is low in both total and saturated fat. Organic costs more but assures you of a quality product that we believe is better for your health and has a far superior taste. The next best option is to choose 'free range' since neither organic nor free range chickens have been fed antibiotics and they have access to an outside run (see page 85-6 for more information).
eggs—free range or organic	Come pretty close to a complete food. Numerous vitamins and minerals (primarily in the yolk). Go for omega-3 enriched. Only 1.5 grams saturated fat per egg so unjustly labelled a 'bad' food.
fish—especially oily	Oily fish are the best source of omega-3 fats crucial for optimal health. All fish is low in saturated fats and contain all essential amino acids. Good source of iodine, iron and zinc (see page 90 for information on mercury in fish).
game meats, for example kangaroo and venison	Incredibly lean, very low in saturated fat and provide omega-3 fats while providing all essential amino acids. Great for iron and zinc. What's more here in Australia, kangaroo, despite being one of the healthiest meats you can buy, is also one of the cheapest.
lean pork	A fabulous source of protein with very little total or saturated fat. Not as good as red meat for iron, but provides good levels of zinc and is a particularly good source of thiamin.
lean red meat	Low in saturated fats. Contains all essential amino acids. Excellent source of iron and zinc in particular. Look for grass-fed rather than grain-fed for lower fat and higher omega-3 levels.
liver	Hard to beat for iron. Excellent source of vitamin A, vitamin C, riboflavin, niacin, vitamin B6, folate, vitamin B12, pantothenic acid, phosphorus, copper and selenium. Good source of zinc. Contains all essential amino acids. Chicken liver has less total and saturated fat than lamb. High in cholesterol therefore limit if you have high blood cholesterol. Be aware that liver products such as pâté are usually very high in fat, much of it saturated from added butter or lard.
low-fat milk and yoghurt	Highest dietary source of calcium. Provides low natural GI carbohydrates. Good source of phosphorus and B group vitamins. Probiotic yoghurts may help with digestive processes.
seafood (excluding prawns, squid and fish roe)	Good source of omega-3 fats and low in saturated fats. Fantastic levels of zinc and iron. Good source of potassium, phosphorus and magnesium.

STAR PERFORMERS

Protein Source	Nutrient Summary
cheeses naturally lower in fat, for example, ricotta, cottage	Excellent source of calcium and provide all essential amino acids. Low-fat dairy foods have been shown in some studies to assist in weight loss, possibly due to high levels of the amino acid leucine present. No need to buy the diet versions, the small amount of fat in the regular varieties is fine as part of a healthy diet and they taste immeasurably better.
legumes and pulses	Listed as 5-star performers for carbohydrates, but can't here as they lack one or more of the essential amino acids. Nevertheless, combined with other plant proteins, this is easily overcome and therefore an essential addition to the vegetarian diet. Good plant source of iron.
natural yoghurt (full fat)	Contains the saturated fat found in whole milk, but excellent source of calcium and has no added sugar, additives or flavours. Eaten in moderation the fat is not a problem and does contain fat-soluble vitamins such as A and D.
prawns, squid and fish roe	All the benefits of other seafood but is high in cholesterol. For most this is not a problem, but if you have high blood cholesterol you should limit your intake of these foods to no more than once a week.
smoked fish	All the benefits of fish and with the longer shelf life, provides a convenient source of omega-3 fats. But high sodium content of smoked fish prevents it making the 5-star category. Those with high blood pressure should limit intake. If your sodium intake is otherwise low, smoked fish can happily be included.
soy	Plant source of protein that comes closest to matching the profile of amino acids from animal produce. Excellent therefore for vegetarians. Low in saturated fat. High in antioxidants and phytoestrogens. High intake related to low levels of certain cancers in Asia, but concerns over potential increase in cancer risk with high phytoestrogen intake, particularly from soy supplements. Can reduce LDL-cholesterol levels and reduce risk of heart disease. Bottom line is choose natural soy foods such as tofu, and not processed foods based on soy or supplements (see pages 99–101).

The table below summarises the attributes of each of our protein players including key nutrients, fats present, processing factors and any additional information of note.

Protein Source	Nutrient Summary	
organic low-fat sausages and burger patties	The organic label means more than the source of the meat—it also means that no artificial flavours, additives or preservatives are added. The shelf life will therefore be shorter but the quality immeasurably higher. Look for those with a high meat content and lower in fat.	**GOOD PERFORMERS**
textured vegetable protein (TVP)	TVP is basically defatted soya flour that has been processed and dried to give a substance with a sponge-like texture which may be flavoured to resemble meat. Used in products such as vegetarian sausages. Nutritionally, it provides a good source of plant protein with very little fat but, at the end of the day, it is a manufactured and processed product and as such not a star performing player in our book.	
veal	Veal is defined as meat from a calf up to six months old. In Europe, the abysmal treatment of animals continues (despite aggressive lobbying from animal welfare groups) as this produces the very white meat prized particularly by French cuisine. Animals are individually penned to restrict movement and deprived of iron and sunshine. In Australia, this should not happen. Generally, animals are penned in groups of 8-10 and are fed a combination of milk and grains. The result is a more pink meat. However, the RSPCA report that not all producers are heeding animal welfare issues and, for this reason, we cannot include veal as a star performer. Nutritionally it is very lean and low in saturated fat and, while not so high in iron as red meat, it is a good source of zinc and other nutrients.	
chicken thigh, leg or wing	More fat, especially saturated fat than breast meat. At home, remove the skin and any visible fat. Does contain more iron than breast meat.	**RESERVES**
duck and goose	Fattier meats with a high proportion of saturated fat. You can significantly reduce this by removing the skin.	
fatty cuts of red meat	Significant source of saturated fat in Western diets. Watch out for grain-fed meats that may not have a visible layer of fat, but marbling where the fat is throughout the meat and impossible to remove.	
full fat cheese	Delicious to us cheese lovers but very high saturated fat content. You don't need to avoid it, just exercise moderation and enjoy a small serve. Undeniably great for calcium and good for your teeth when consumed at the end of a meal. Another dietary habit the French have gotten right!	
flavoured yoghurts (low and full fat)	All have added sugar and the low-fat versions are often the worst culprits. They also use gums and other additives in an attempt to replace the creamy feel. Full-fat, all-natural varieties are a better option but do contain more kilojoules. Ideally buy natural yoghurt and add your own fruit purée.	
full fat milk	Significant source of saturated fat if you drink a fair bit—a few regular lattés in the day adds up to a lot of milk. Kids under 2 years need the extra nutrition in whole milk, the rest of us benefit from skipping the fat.	
reduced-fat and manufactured low-fat cheese	Less fat but also less taste. This means you're not really satisfied and either eat more or seek another food to eat as well. Choose the real thing but exercise moderation.	
commercial burgers and sausages	Made from the cheapest cuts of meat, full of fat especially saturated fat, and usually fried adding to the risk of trans fats being present. Artificial additives, flavours and preservatives are almost always added. Make your own at home using good quality meat or choose organic low-fat versions instead.	**LIABILITIES**
cured meats, for example prosciutto and bacon	High saturated fat, high sodium and heavily processed.	
diet yoghurts	Artificial sweeteners may not have been proven to do us any harm but are clearly not real natural food. Diet products leave us unsatisfied and usually we seek out more pleasurable food. Avoid anything labelled 'diet'.	
salami	The solid fat you can see in lumps is saturated fat. Also high in sodium and preservatives commonly used.	

Chapter 5

Fats

For over two decades, health authorities around the world have recommended that we follow a low-fat diet. This was touted as the best way to lose weight and reduce your risk of heart disease. Many of us sat up and listened and did our best to comply. Food manufacturers did their part and produced a plethora of low-fat foods, including low-fat versions of many of our favourites which would otherwise be banished from a low-fat diet. We can now buy low- or at least reduced-fat biscuits, cakes, milk, cheese, burgers, sausages, margarine, and even chocolate! The message that choosing these foods over their high-fat counterparts will do us good had been little questioned—until now.

While apparent intakes of fat have been declining in Australia, and in most countries in the developed world, overweight and obesity rates continue to rise at an alarming rate. Something is clearly going wrong. There are three alternative views of what that is:

1. Fat intakes are not really declining—it just appears that way from the methods used in dietary surveys. While many of us have made the switch to low-fat milk and choose lower fat products, we also consume more 'hidden' fat in fast food, restaurant and takeaway meals, and in luxury goods and treats such as ice cream, desserts and confectionery.

2. Fat intakes have truly declined but what we are replacing the fat with is just as bad, if not worse, than what we were eating before. We eat more and more processed food that tends to provide the worst types of carbohydrate (high GI), low levels of nutrients and fibre and, despite their low fat content, they have a high energy density. In other words, they pack a lot of kilojoules into each gram. While they are low in fat, they are not low kilojoule.

3. The recommendations were wrong and lowering your fat intake does not in fact improve weight control over the long term.

There is evidence to support each of these three seemingly opposing views and they may all be right, or at least all be contributing to the problem. The latest reports from large-scale studies in the US have failed to show that reducing the fat intake of your diet long term has any beneficial outcome on overweight, weight gain, heart disease or cancer (Beresford et al, 2006; Howard et al, 2006a; Howard et al, 2006b; Prentice et al, 2006). However, what these studies have shown is that it is not the total amount of fat that is important, but the type of fat that you eat. In short, bad fats increase your risk of heart disease and certain other diseases, while good fats lower the risk.

This explanation fits with all three of the views above. If view 1 is correct and we are simply eating our fat from different sources, then we are likely to be eating more of the bad fats and less of the good. If view 2 is correct we are reducing our intake of all fats, including the good ones now known to reduce our risk of disease. And view 3 is directly backed up by this research, suggesting recommendations to reduce total fat intake may be out of date.

This new research makes sense when we think of two of the healthiest known diets on earth: the Japanese diet with a very low fat content of 20 per cent; and the Mediterranean diet with a relatively high fat intake of up to 40 per cent. Both of these regions have low rates of heart disease which can't be explained by total fat intake. However, they do have several things in common, one of which is that both contain good levels of healthy fats and low levels of the bad fats. So what makes a fat good or bad?

The best fats will	FATS	The worst fats will
✓ contain predominately the good unsaturated fats		✗ contain high levels of saturated and/or trans fats
✓ may also be a good source of the essential omega-3 fats		✗ raise blood levels of 'bad' LDL cholesterol
✓ be rich in other essential nutrients such as fat-soluble vitamins A, D or E, and/or antioxidants		✗ increase our risk of chronic disease including heart disease and certain cancers
✓ Increase blood levels of 'good' HDL cholesterol, while lowering 'bad' LDL cholesterol		✗ may be stored more readily as body fat and burned less readily as fuel
✓ reduce our risk of chronic disease including heart disease and certain cancers		✗ be accompanied by non-food additives such as preservatives, flavouring and fat-replacers that have little or no nutritional value
✓ may be burned more readily as fuel thus helping us to lose body fat		

FIGURE 5.1 The best and worst of fats

The different types of fats

Fats are made up of individual fatty acids and these can be grouped into three main types—saturated, monounsaturated and polyunsaturated. All fats contain a mixture of these three but will be predominantly of one type; for example, butter contains predominantly saturated fatty acids and therefore we tend to call butter a saturated fat.

The polyunsaturated fats can be further divided into the omega-6 and the omega-3 fats. The ratio between these two types of fats seems to be critical to health and, while in hunter–gatherer days man ate a ratio of close to 1 to 1, today we tend to eat far more omega-6 and not nearly enough omega-3, giving us a ratio closer to 14 to 1! The amount of each type of fat in common oils and fats is shown in Figure 5.2.

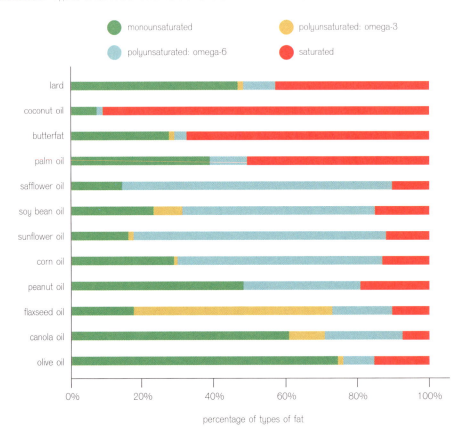

FIGURE 5.2 Types of fat in common oils and fats

A further type of fat is trans fat. Although very small amounts of trans fats do occur in natural foods, dietary intakes have dramatically increased due to our greater consumption of processed foods. Trans fats are produced during the chemical process called hydrogenation, that turns a liquid oil into a solid. This was originally done in the production of margarine, but now hydrogenated oils are used widely in the commercial production of biscuits, cakes, doughnuts, pastry, fast foods and so on. In fact many of today's margarines boast 'virtually no trans fats' while consumers are unaware of the significant levels in some of these other foods.

So which are bad fats and which are good?

Primarily, this is based on how the fat affects blood LDL and HDL-cholesterol levels. A high level of LDL-cholesterol can result in it being taken up into the walls of the coronary arteries—this is part of the process of atherosclerosis which narrows the arteries and increases the risk of having a heart attack. A high level of HDL-cholesterol on the other hand is protective against heart disease since it is involved in transporting cholesterol back to the liver for elimination from the body. In general, therefore, the lowest risk of heart disease comes from low 'bad' LDL-cholesterol and high 'good' HDL-cholesterol levels in the blood.

BAD FATS

Saturated and trans fats both raise LDL-cholesterol levels and are therefore targeted as the fats we need to reduce in our diet. However *trans fats are the worst of all*. While saturated fats raise good HDL-cholesterol levels as well as the bad LDL, trans fats *lower* good HDL-cholesterol while raising bad LDL. A key step to improving your health is to avoid these fats wherever possible. For this reason, we have ranked foods containing hydrogenated, or partially hydrogenated, oils as liabilities.

While most fat research has centred on heart disease and the effects of fats on blood cholesterol, there has started to be more interest on how fats may be metabolised differently and therefore contribute more or less to body fat stores.

While the research is in the early days and by no means conclusive, there is the suggestion that, compared to unsaturated fats, saturated fat may be stored more readily and burned as fuel less readily. In other words, is saturated fat more fattening than other fats? Since technically all fats contain the same kilojoules per gram this is a controversial idea, but given that this fits in nicely with the conclusions from the heart disease research, it can only compound the recommendations to reduce our intake of saturated fat.

GOOD FATS

Essentially, all unsaturated fats are good fats since they improve blood cholesterol levels; raising good HDL-cholesterol and reducing bad LDL-cholesterol. If you don't consume these fats and instead follow the traditional advice to eat a low-fat diet, you still reduce bad LDL-cholesterol but you also lower good HDL-cholesterol. This is undoubtedly part of the explanation as to why low-fat diets have produced such disappointing results in the long-term studies previously mentioned.

The omega-3 polyunsaturated fats deserve a special mention since they seem to be particularly important to health:

★ Omega-3 fats can **reduce your risk of cardiovascular disease** in three ways—by 'thinning' the blood making it less likely that a clot will form and result in a heart attack; by protecting the heart from potentially fatal rhythm disturbances; and by improving the function of the blood vessels thus reducing blood pressure. Certainly for those with existing heart disease, consuming more omega-3 fats is arguably one of the most important nutrition changes you can make. A large European study found that in volunteers who had already had one heart attack, those who took an omega-3 supplement reduced their risk of dying from heart disease by 25 per cent (GISSI-Prevenzione Investigators, 1999).

★ Omega-3 fats have an **anti-inflammatory** effect in the body and are therefore also useful in treating (and possibly preventing) disorders that involve inflammation such as arthritis, inflammatory bowel disease and skin disorders including psoriasis, eczema and acne.

★ Omega-3 fats are known to be **crucial for brain development and function**. In fact, brain tissue from humans and animals has been shown to have very high levels of omega-3s. In babies and young children, omega-3s have been linked to development and IQ. Interestingly, breast milk contains these essential fats while formula milks do not unless specifically fortified. Perhaps this explains some of the findings regarding childhood IQ and infant feeding practices. However, we also know that omega-3s continue to be important for the brain into adulthood and have even been shown to be helpful in treating some forms of depression.

★ Omega-3 fats have a role in the functioning of the **eye** and recent research suggests they may be protective against macular degeneration, a major cause of blindness worldwide.

★ Omega-3 fats may be important for a **strong immune system** and may even protect against some forms of cancer.

★ Omega-3 fats may even assist in promoting **fat burning** and improving body composition when combined with exercise. This was shown in a recent Australian study that reported a surprise result where the combination of a fish oil supplement combined with exercise resulted in a 5 per cent loss of body fat—an effect not seen in either treatment alone (Hill et al, 2007). While needing more research to back this up, this is an exciting result as it corresponded with an increased burning of fat during the exercise showing us that the type of fat, and not just the amount, you eat has an impact on your level of body fat.

In boosting your intake of omega-3 fats, it is important to make sure you are not simultaneously taking in too many omega-6 fats, since these will limit your ability to absorb and utilise the omega-3s. This is one reason why it is a good idea to use a monounsaturated fat, such as olive oil, for basic use rather than using polyunsaturated fats such as sunflower oil.

How much omega-3?

How much omega-3 you need in your diet really depends on the results you want. If you have an inflammatory condition that may be helped by an increased amount of omega-3 you probably need to take a supplement, unless you are prepared to eat a lot of fish and seafood. However, be careful with supplements as too much omega-3 can cause bleeding problems. Always make sure you tell your doctor about any supplements you take as, particularly if you are also on medications, these can interact with seemingly innocuous dietary supplements. For this reason, the US Food and Drug Administration recommends that consumers not exceed more than a total of 3 grams per day, with no more than 2 grams per day from a dietary supplement. Here in Australia the most recent dietary recommendations from the National Health and Medical Research Council (NHMRC) suggest a daily intake of long chain omega-3 fats of 430 milligrams for women and 610 milligrams for men to reduce the risk of

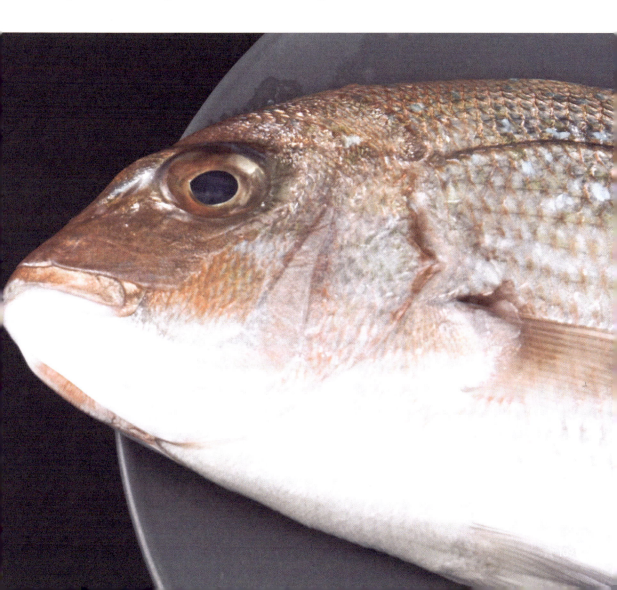

chronic disease. To give you an idea of how much fish you need to eat to achieve these targets, Table 5.1 shows the omega-3 content per 100 grams in descending order of typical Australian fish and seafood. Swordfish is the resounding winner with over 1000 milligrams, so it is a real shame this fish is also one most likely to be contaminated with mercury and it is an unsustainable fish. Have it no more than once a week to be on the safe side.

TABLE 5.1 Omega-3 content per 100 grams of selected Australian fish and seafood (Nichols et al, 1998)

Fish	Seafood
Swordfish 1059 milligrams	Krill (average 2 varieties) 482 milligrams
Atlantic salmon 689 milligrams	Sydney rock oyster 397 milligrams
Mackerel (average of 3 varieties) 461 milligrams	Blue mussel 389 milligrams
Gemfish 441 milligrams	Squid 362 milligrams
Queensland mullet 405 milligrams	Pacific oyster 325 milligrams
Silver perch 386 milligrams	Scallop 321 milligrams
Australian herring 370 milligrams	Calamari 304 milligrams
Yellowtail kingfish 322 milligrams	Blue swimmer crab 249 milligrams
Australian salmon (average of 3 varieties) 321 milligrams	Baby octopus 214 milligrams
Rainbow trout 309 milligrams	Pipi 170 milligrams
Sardines (average of 2 varieties) 252 milligrams	Eastern king prawn 151 milligrams
Southern bluefin tuna 224 milligrams	Western king prawn 126 milligrams
Snapper 223 milligrams	Tiger prawn (average of 3 varieties) 114 milligrams
Red mullet 218 milligrams	Rock lobster (average of 4 varieties) 106 milligrams
Flathead (average of 6 varieties) 200 milligrams	Mud crab 89 milligrams
John dory 188 milligrams	Yabby 69 milligrams
Silver trevally 182 milligrams	Moreton Bay bug 68 milligrams
King George whiting 123 milligrams	
Yellowfin tuna 117 milligrams	
Ling 113 milligrams	
Barramundi (average of fresh- & saltwater) 94 milligrams	

It might look as though you need to eat fish every day to reach the recommended omega-3 intake, but remember you also get these fats in many other foods including meat, enriched eggs, linseed, canola, walnut and mustard oils, leafy greens and omega-3 enriched products (see Table 5.2). To meet the target, most heart disease associations around the world recommend at least two fish meals a week, but see this as the minimum. If you can, aim for three to five fish meals per week. This might sound a lot, but remember that canned and packet fish also counts, so fish meals can include tuna/salmon in your sandwich. This, then is not so hard to achieve. With a little thought and planning you can achieve an omega-3-rich diet.

TABLE 5.2 Types of fat in food

GOOD FATS   # BAD FATS

Monounsaturated fats	Polyunsaturated fats		Saturated fats	Trans fats
	omega-3s	omega-6s		
olive oil	oily fish, for example, salmon, trout, sardines, mackerel, herring	seeds and seed oils including sunflower, safflower and sesame (tahini)	butter	stick margarines (solid like butter)
canola oil	seafood including mussels, oysters, calamari and octopus	corn oil	visible fat on meat	commercially baked products including biscuits, cakes, doughnuts and pastries
peanuts, peanut oil and peanut butter	linseed oil (flaxseed)	soy bean oil	meat products, for example sausages, burgers and salami	commercial deep-fried foods, for example many fast foods
pecans	sesame seeds, tahini and hummus	soft tub margarines made from the oils	palm oil	shortening
pistachios	walnuts and walnut oil	walnuts	full-fat milk	
cashews	meat from grass-fed animals	Brazil nuts	cheese	
hazelnuts	leafy green vegetables	pine nuts	lard	
almonds	omega-3 enriched eggs		coconut and coconut oil*	
macadamias	krill (small shrimp-like crustaceans)			
	wakame (seaweed used widely in Japanese cooking)			

* rich in saturated fats of medium chain length which are not cholesterol-raising and have many potential benefits. See page 123 for more information.

Butter or margarine?

Life used to be simple. You spread butter on your bread, melted it over vegetables and used it in cooking. The biggest decision you had to make was which of a handful of brands to buy. Then new research discovered that saturated fat raises our cholesterol and increases our risk of heart disease. Over 65 per cent of the fat in butter is saturated. Very quickly butter topped the 'bad food' list and we searched for an alternative. Margarine, originally produced as a cheap spread, was suddenly promoted as the healthy choice and sales quickly overtook those for butter. But it all went wrong when scientists discovered that the chemical process used to turn an oil into a spread, created a type of fat called trans fat that was even worse for us than saturated fat. Fast forward to today and the debate continues to rage as to which is the healthier choice—butter or margarine?

The use of butter can be traced as far back as 2000 BC and there are numerous references to

Butter or margarine? (continued)

the food in the Bible. What could be a more humble but delicious meal than bread and butter? In contrast, margarine was invented as a substitute for butter by a Frenchman in 1870, although only became widely popular during and after the war years. Today margarine sales far outweigh butter in most Western countries, largely due to the perceived health benefits. But can a modern manufactured product, which goes against the nutrition purist's idea of eating food as close to nature as possible, really be healthier than the fat made from churning wholesome cow's milk? As passionate believers in eating 'real' foods as much as possible, we have to confess to struggling with the idea that we can manufacture something that is better for us than a relatively simple food that has been made and consumed by native communities for thousands of years. But we'll give you the facts and you can make up your own mind.

From a nutritional point of view there is no doubt of the winner. The saturated fat in butter is not good for us since it tends to raise 'bad' LDL-cholesterol in blood, increasing our risk of heart disease. On the other hand, manufacturers of margarines responded quickly to the new information on trans fats and produced a new generation of margarines with little or none. If you read the labels of the vast majority of margarines on today's supermarket shelves you'll be hard pushed to find any with a significant level of trans fats. The only ones to watch out for are harder stick varieties of margarine. Oils are liquid at room temperature; therefore, the harder the margarine is, the greater the likelihood the fats have been hydrogenated. The fat in margarines comes predominately from the oils used to make the spread—canola, sunflower, olive, soy and so on—and as a result they are high in healthy mono- and poly-unsaturated fats. These fats have the ability to lower 'bad' LDL-cholesterol. In fact a US study of 46 families published in the *Journal of the American Medical Association* found that substituting margarine for butter successfully lowered blood cholesterol levels (Denke et al, 2000).

Plant sterol margarines take this a step further. Plant sterols bind cholesterol in the gut (from both food and cholesterol excreted in bile acids as part of the digestive process) preventing it from being re-absorbed. Studies have shown that these margarines can be extremely effective in lowering blood cholesterol. There is no doubt that if you have pre-existing high cholesterol levels, using a plant sterol margarine can help and, if this reduces the need for cholesterol-lowering drugs, this has to be a good thing. The only catch is you have to make sure you use enough of it—a fairly generous spread on 3–4 slices of bread—and it is more expensive. Other margarines have omega-3 fats from fish added—these are fats that there is little doubt we no longer eat enough of. Yet you could just choose to eat fish and/or seafood more often. For those that can't or won't, such margarines provide some benefit.

For the butter lovers, take heart that butter does contain several essential nutrients—in particular the fat-soluble vitamins A, D and E. Margarines are fortified with these nutrients to match the composition of butter. During our phase of obsession over reducing fat, these nutrients have been neglected. So, if you love butter, the answer is just don't have too much of it! Enjoy a little on your bread or a skim on your toast in the morning, but use healthier alternatives the rest of the time.

Butter or margarine? We're going to play the devil's advocate and suggest neither. Butter is clearly not the best sort of fat for our heart health. Margarine is a modern invention and not a part of our ancestors' or native traditional diets around the world. After all, an olive oil margarine is not the same as a Mediterranean-style olive oil-based diet, and an omega-3-enriched margarine is not the same as a diet high in fish and seafood. So instead brush your bread with olive oil, use a nut spread on toast, use mashed avocado in sandwiches and cook with olive or other healthy oils.

A note for cheese lovers

Cheese in general is an energy-dense food due to its high fat and low water content, and as such can contribute to overweight if you indulge too much. This, together with the fact that it is a significant source of saturated fat, has earned it a bad name. However, there are many good attributes to cheese. It contains all of the essential amino acids and therefore is a great source of protein; it is one of the richest food sources of calcium; it also provides other essential nutrients including vitamin A, phosphorus and zinc; and when eaten at the end of a meal cheese is good for your teeth by providing a pool of minerals surrounding the tooth enamel.

The bottom line, therefore, is you can include cheese happily in your diet if you wish, but just watch how much. Ending a meal with an enormous cheese platter with biscuits is not the best plan for health—save that for an occasional treat. Using strong cheese is generally a good idea as you'll tend to use less, and you can also choose cheeses with a lower saturated fat content for more regular use. The fat contents of the various cheeses are shown in Table 5.3.

TABLE 5.3 Comparing the total and saturated fat content in 30 grams of different cheeses

Type of cheese	Fat (grams)	Saturated fat (grams)
cottage cheese	1.7	1.1
ricotta cheese	3.4	2.2
reduced-fat feta	4.3	2.8
bocconcini	4.6	3.0
goat's cheese	4.7	3.1
light Philadelphia cream cheese	5.0	3.3
haloumi	5.1	3.3
mozzarella	6.6	4.2
reduced-fat (−25 per cent) cheddar	7.1	4.5
feta	7.0	4.6
camembert	7.9	5.1
brie	8.7	5.6
Swiss cheese	9.0	5.7
blue vein cheese and Parmesan	9.7	6.2
Philadelphia cream cheese	9.9	6.4
cheddar (mild, tasty, vintage)	10.1	6.5

Choosing the right oil

Further confusion over which oil to use occurs when you consider the extraction process and what you intend to do with the oil. The 5-star performing flaxseed oil can be relegated to the liabilities if you decide to use it in the deep-fat fryer!

The smoke point of oil is the temperature it can reach before it starts to break down. Heating an oil to the point of smoking will affect the taste and increase the risk of carcinogens on the cooked food. Most unrefined oils have a relatively low smoke point. Refined oils on the other hand have a much higher smoke point but the methods used to refine sometimes include numerous health-devaluing processes including bleaching, deodorising and de-gumming. Oils are generally refined unless otherwise stipulated on the bottle. The term cold pressed means a naturally extracted oil using gentle low temperature extraction methods. Extra virgin is the name applied to the first batch of oil extracted directly from the fruit, nut or seed. Oils that are predominantly polyunsaturated can easily become rancid when exposed to heat, light and oxygen and the processing methods may accelerate this transition. The price of the oil is therefore a good determinant of the quality of oil. Cheaper oils are typically produced through a mass chemical refining and extraction process and while they have a high smoke point they can ultimately be as bad for the health as cooking in lard. A safeguard from buying oil extracted and refined through a myriad of chemicals is to buy organic. For a product to receive organic certification, the entire process must be approved by the Australian Quarantine and Inspection service. Of all products used in the processing, 95 per cent must be organic with the remaining 5 per cent used from traditional natural ingredients free of synthetic flavours or chemicals.

An easy guide to selecting oils

- Where no heat is required, the healthiest oils are cold pressed extra virgin.
- Where moderate heat is required, select unrefined oils that can withstand the heat (see cooking guide).
- Where the highest cooking temperatures are required, select refined organic oils.

Do

★ Stock a maximum of four oils at any one time.

★ Buy smaller bottles and use them quickly.

★ Store oils in the fridge or cool dark cupboard.

★ Buy oils in dark glass bottles.

★ Check expiry date and throw out old oils that may be rancid.

Don't

★ Re-use oil.

★ Store expensive oils for special occasions—enjoy them straight away.

★ Heat oils to their smoke point.

★ Have dozens of oils for every occasion—it's better to have a few all-purpose oils and replace them regularly.

TABLE 5.4 Cooking guide for oils

Cooking application

	Smoke point (°C)	Cold use <107°C	Light grilling and gentle frying 107–175°C	Medium frying and baking 175–200°C	Deep-fry, stir-fry, barbecue >200°C	Notes
UNREFINED						
Almond	221	•	•	•	•	Expensive oil for regular use—use in cold desserts or salad dressings. Use it quickly to prevent it becoming rancid.
Avocado	250	•	•	•	•	Delicious and healthy but is expensive. Heavy flavoured.
Camellia tea	195	•	•	•		Excellent flavoured viscous oil for frying and baking.
Canola	107	•				Not a great choice when there are so many traditional, better flavoured oils available.
Corn	160	•	•			A soft sweet brightly coloured oil.
Coconut	176	•	•	•		Used extensively in Asian cooking.
Flaxseed	107	•				Delicious nutty-flavoured oil for salad dressings. Is highly unstable and therefore must *never* be heated.
Hazelnut	221	•			•	Like all nut oils it's an expensive oil for everyday use. Use it quickly to prevent it becoming rancid.
Grapeseed	215	•	•			Light flavoured and suitable for most cooking and baking. Makes a good base for a salad dressing where the oil carries other flavours rather than being the base.
Macadamia	198	•				Like all nut oils it's an expensive oil for everyday use. Use it quickly to prevent it becoming rancid.
Olive, cold pressed	160	•	•			Best drizzled over salads and as replacement for butter with bread.
Olive, extra virgin	205	•	•	•		Good all-purpose oil for moderate heat cooking.
Olive, virgin	215	•	•	•	•	Good all-purpose staple for everything.
Peanut	160	•	•			Buy organic as a safeguard against toxins.
Safflower	107	•				Light flavoured oil for salad dressing.
Sesame	176	•	•			Strong flavoured oil, can be added for flavour after cooking stir-fries and other Asian dishes
Sunflower	107	•				Light flavoured oil for salad dressing.
Sunflower, high oleic	160	•	•			Available from health food stores. The higher smoke point allows it be to used for light cooking purposes.
Walnut	160	•	•			Delicious oil for dressing and low temperature cooking.
REFINED						
Avocado	270	•	•	•	•	Look for organic refined oils which have not gone through an extensive chemical refining process. Select them for preferred flavour.
Camellia Tea	220	•	•	•	•	
Canola Oil	210	•	•	•	•	
Corn	210	•	•	•	•	
Grapeseed	251	•	•	•	•	
Olive	242	•	•	•	•	
Peanut	226	•	•	•	•	
Safflower	265	•	•	•	•	
Sesame	232	•	•	•	•	
Soy	250	•	•	•	•	
Sunflower	232	•	•	•	•	
Sunflower, high oleic	232	•	•	•	•	
Walnut	204	•	•	•		

Ranking the Players – Fats

Rolling out the fat players – no pun intended!

Each player was assigned a division based on its nutritional profile. The criteria for the selection process were based on their ability to protect and maintain a healthy body for optimal performance. Consideration was given to the quality and type of fat, key nutrients, antioxidants/phytochemicals and processing factors.

STAR PERFORMERS

Fat Source
coconut and coconut oil
macadamias
peanuts, peanut butter and unrefined peanut oil

5-STAR PERFORMERS

Fat Source	
avocado and unrefined avocado oil	
camellia tea oil	
linseeds (flaxseeds) and linseed oil	
Nuts and seeds	almonds, Brazil nuts, cashews, hazelnuts, nut spreads/butters, pecans, pine nuts, pistachios, sesame seeds and tahini (sesame butter), sunflower seeds, walnuts
oily fish including Atlantic salmon, trout, silver perch, sardines, mackerel, herring and Queensland mullet	
olives and unrefined olive oil	
seafood including oysters, mussels, squid, calamari, octopus	

GOOD PERFORMERS

unrefined grapeseed oil
unrefined sesame oil
unrefined sunflower oil and safflower oil
whole-egg fresh mayonnaise

RESERVES

butter
canola oil
corn oil
full-fat dairy products
monounsaturated margarines, for example olive oil spread
plant sterol margarines
refined oils
rice bran oil
roasted salted nuts including peanuts
soy bean oil

LIABILITIES

commercially baked products including doughnuts, cakes, pastries and biscuits	
commercially deep-fried food and fast food	
commercial mayonnaise	salad dressing (cream)
lard	shortening
low- and reduced-fat spreads	stick/block margarines
palm oil	suet and tallow
polyunsaturated margarines	visible meat fat

5-star performers for fats

AVOCADO AND AVOCADO OIL

Avocados contain over 25 essential nutrients including potassium, magnesium, B group vitamins, folate and vitamin C. Avocados were for a long time on the dieter's list of 'foods to avoid' due to their high fat content. Thankfully, we now know better and the type of fat found in avocados is predominately healthy monounsaturated fat. The presence of fat also means that avocados are a source of the fat-soluble vitamin and important antioxidant, vitamin E. Furthermore if you add avocado to a salad or sandwich, the fat will then enable your body to absorb the carotenoids, and many other nutrients, found in the other plant foods. These are fat soluble and so if you only ever eat low-fat salads and dressings you absorb very few of these powerful antioxidants. Avocados contain several other disease-fighting phytochemicals including glutathione, involved in detoxification and antioxidant systems in the body; beta-sitosterol, which reduces blood cholesterol levels; and lutein, a carotenoid antioxidant thought to play an important role in eye health, preventing age-related macular degeneration, and in protecting the skin from sun damage.

Avocado oil may be new to you, but it is well worth seeking out. Look for one that is cold pressed and unrefined and you have an oil that preserves the nutrients and antioxidants found in the fat component of the raw fruit. The oil is very high in monounsaturated fat and very low in saturated fat making it pretty ideal from a nutritional perspective. It also has the advantage of a higher smoke point than olive oil, making it an excellent choice for sautéing, stir-frying and pan-frying.

CAMELLIA TEA OIL

Another oil new to our shores, yet one which has been used in Asian countries for thousands of years, is camellia tea oil (not to be confused with tea tree oil). The oil, extracted from the seeds of the camellia tea bush grown in the mountains of China has, like avocado oil, the advantage both in its refined and unrefined state of possessing a high smoke point, making it suitable for most cooking applications. It is said to be 97 per cent digestible and used in traditional Chinese medicine to strengthen the spleen. With over 80 per cent of its fat content from monounsaturated fat—even higher than olive oil—camellia tea oil is extremely stable and can assist in lowering high levels of 'bad' LDL-cholesterol and reduce the risk of heart disease. It's another great source of the antioxidant vitamin E and provides the omega-9 family of fats, currently being researched for their effect on various inflammatory processes in the body. Refined camellia tea oil is organic and therefore free of any residual chemicals used during the extraction process. The oil has a unique smoky flavour and is delicious in salad dressings, stir-fries and even served with wholegrain sourdough bread.

NUTS AND SEEDS

As with avocados, nuts and seeds were once admonished, particularly as part of weight-control diets, due to their high fat and energy content. Yet research shows that not only do regular nut eaters tend to have lower body weights, they also have less cardiovascular disease.

Nuts and seeds provide a good plant source of protein, making them particularly beneficial additions to vegetarian diets. Nuts provide many other essential nutrients to benefit our overall health. They are good for our bones providing magnesium—30 grams of Brazil nuts provides about a third of our daily needs—and small amounts of calcium, particularly almonds. They provide iron and zinc, two minerals often low in our diet, particularly if you don't eat meat. Cashews are the clear winners here with 30 grams providing women with 8 per cent of daily iron and 21 per cent of daily zinc needs (19 per cent and 12 per cent respectively for men). Nuts also provide a whole battery of B group vitamins necessary to convert the food we eat into energy for the body, for healthy skin, hair and nails, and to maintain healthy blood cells.

One large US study found that eating a small handful of nuts (30 grams) on five or more days a week, halved the risk of heart disease! Even those who ate nuts once a week had less heart disease than those who rarely ate nuts (Fraser et al, 1992). Pecans, pistachios, cashews, almonds and hazelnuts provide predominantly monounsaturated fat, while Brazil nuts, walnuts, pine nuts, and sunflower and sesame seeds are all rich in polyunsaturated fats. These fats have been shown to help lower 'bad' LDL-cholesterol levels in the blood, while raising 'good' HDL-cholesterol. There are even some super-healthy omega-3 fats in good quantities in pecans, walnuts and hazelnuts. But it's not just the fat. Nuts provide a whole host of essential nutrients that benefit the heart. Nuts are fibre-rich and this undoubtedly contributes to the cholesterol-lowering effect of nuts. They also provide protein and, in particular, the amino acid arginine known to be important in maintaining healthy blood flow through the arteries. Antioxidants are a major part of our defence against damaged, clogged arteries and nuts are full of them. These include vitamin E—almonds are a particularly good source of this vitamin with a small handful providing 80 per cent of the daily needs of men and 100 per cent those of women—as well as lesser known, but just as important, antioxidants including flavonoids, carotenoids and phenolic compounds. In a study of total antioxidant power in different plant foods, walnuts ranked particularly high. Two to three Brazil nuts are all you need to meet your daily requirement for selenium. This mineral plays a vital antioxidant role in preventing cellular damage and is crucial for healthy immune and thyroid function.

Eating nuts may also help you to control your weight in two ways. First, nuts are very satiating and successfully curb our hunger and desire to eat. By eating nuts we avoid overeating other (probably less nutritious) foods. Second, nuts are an intact food containing lots of fibre— the body has to work hard to break down the individual cell walls to absorb and make use of the energy and nutrients. This in turn may mean that we are not 100 per cent successful in completing the task and therefore fail to absorb all of the energy, particularly from fat, contained in the nut. In other words we may be getting fewer kilojoules and fat from nuts than predicted from the nutrient composition data.

To get the most from these 5-star performing foods, steer clear of the salted roasted varieties and the nut butters with added sugar, salt, other additives and preservatives. Buy your nuts raw and unsalted—you can roast them yourself for a few minutes in a hot oven—and as natural, unadulterated butters. You'll find these in the health food section of your supermarket and they are delicious on toast instead of butter.

LINSEED (flaxseed) AND LINSEED OIL

Linseeds (sometimes called flaxseeds) deserve a separate mention as they are fairly unique in providing a good plant source of omega-3 fats. They are not quite the same as the ones you find in oily fish and seafood, they are the shorter chain versions from the same fat family and can be elongated in the body to produce the beneficial long chain ones. There is little doubt that regularly consuming fish and seafood is the best means of upping your omega-3 intake but, for those who won't or can't, linseeds are the next best thing. Omega-3 fats tend to help reduce inflammatory reactions in the body and this may explain why some studies have shown flaxseeds to be helpful in reducing the painful symptoms of arthritis, gout and inflammatory bowel disease such as Crohn's.

Linseeds are rich in both soluble and insoluble fibre. The soluble fibre helps to reduce cholesterol levels and slow the absorption of carbohydrate from other foods eaten at the same time, resulting in lower glucose and insulin responses. The insoluble fibre is beneficial for the gut, helping to keep you regular, provide a fuel source to beneficial bacteria and keep the colon healthy.

Linseeds also appear to have anti-cancer properties. They are rich in lignans—phytoestrogens similar to those found in soy. These have been shown to reduce cancer risk, particularly cancer of the breast, prostate and possibly colon and skin.

To achieve a therapeutic effect from linseed, you need about 25 grams a day or a tablespoon of linseed oil. The seeds offer the most complete range of benefits and can be ground to form a flour or meal. The flour can be refrigerated for up to three days, and sprinkled over cereal, used with low-fat yoghurt or cottage cheese or added to almost any baked item, including biscuits, breads, muffins or scones at 6–8 per cent of the dry ingredients. Linseed oil has a very low smoke point and should therefore never be heated—use in salad dressings or drizzle over your morning cereal.

OILY FISH

Oily fish are undoubtedly the best food source of omega-3 fats and there is convincing evidence that eating more fish can reduce our risk of cardiovascular disease. If you have existing heart disease, eating more fish is possibly the most important nutritional change you could make. One large Italian trial found that people who had survived a heart attack could lower their risk of dying from a second attack by 25 per cent by consuming 1 gram per day of omega-3 fats (GISSI-Prevenzione Investigators, 1999). In this trial, the participants were given an omega-3 supplement—to reach this level of intake from fish alone would mean eating a serve of oily fish every day. For the rest of us, we needn't consume this much to gain health benefits; the current recommendations are to include at least two servings per week of oily fish.

See page 110 for the omega-3 content of common Australian fish and seafood.

OLIVES AND UNREFINED OLIVE OIL

Olives and olive oil provide the major source of fat in the traditional Mediterranean diet, and the low level of heart disease in this region is thought to be at least in part attributed to this. The fat is predominately monounsaturated fat, which is more stable than polyunsaturated fat, both as a food and once it's ingested and incorporated into cells in the body. It is therefore less susceptible to oxidation and bodily damage. As a food, the oil is less likely to go rancid and, once in the body, is thought to help prevent cancers by resisting the type of free radical damage that instigates the cancer process. Olives and cold pressed olive oil are also rich in phenol compounds that are natural antioxidants. They have been shown to have a number of desirable effects from helping to reduce skin damage from the sun to lowering blood cholesterol levels, blood pressure and the risk of heart disease (Covas et al, 2006). However the phenol content of olive oil is not consistent and many of the mass market oils available in the supermarket will have poor levels. There are differences between olive varieties and whether the olives are picked late or early in the season, but the major effects on phenol content are how the oil is processed and the length of time the oil is subsequently stored. Most of the standard olive oils have been refined—a process involving filtering, charcoal treatment, heating and chemical treatment to adjust acidity—and this dramatically reduces the phenol content. According to the Olive Oil Source (www.oliveoilsource.com), unrefined, cold pressed olive oil contains 50–80 ppm phenols, while refined oil has only 5 ppm. The longer the oil is stored, whether that be in storage tanks at the manufacturing plant or in the bottle in your pantry, the more phenols are slowly oxidised and used up. So, in order to ensure you have an oil with a high antioxidant phenol content, choose a high quality extra virgin olive oil that is from the current harvest season and that has been properly stored. The bottle should be a dark colour to reduce exposure to light and buy in small quantities to reduce storage time.

You may have to look in a quality health food store or deli for the best choice. These contain as many as 5 milligrams of antioxidant phenols in every 10 grams of olive oil. Of course, this type of oil will be more expensive than the supermarket varieties, so keep specifically for dressings and other cold uses. For cooking, a cheaper olive oil is fine and, because of the effects of heat on extra virgin cold pressed oils (see section on cooking with oils page 115), you'll still get the good fats but not such high levels of phenols. Be aware that light olive oils are not lower in kilojoules, but light in flavour for those who do not like a strong olive flavour. These oils are almost always refined oils and, as a consequence, lack the wonderful antioxidants found in the more flavoursome virgin oils.

SEAFOOD

While oily fish is more usually credited for its omega-3 content, seafood can be equally rich. See page 110 to compare the omega-3 content of popular Australian fish and seafood, and page 98 for general nutritional information on these nutrient-packed foods.

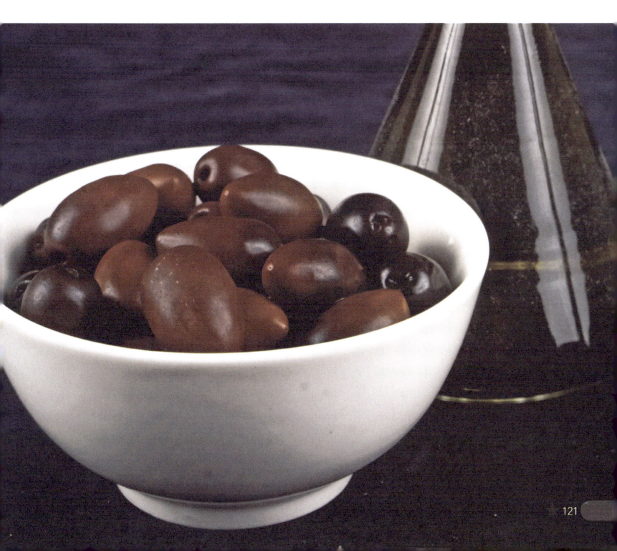

Player Profiles – Fats

5-STAR PERFORMERS

Fat Source	Nutrient Summary
almonds	Good source of calcium and protein, fibre rich and good source of many micronutrients including folate, iron and zinc.
avocado and unrefined avocado oil	The fruit is fibre-rich and provides many additional micronutrients including potassium, magnesium, folate and vitamin C. Avocado oil has a very high smoke point and is therefore a great choice for cooking. It is quite expensive but this is definitely a case for quality over quantity. Use it sparingly and a little will go a long way.
Brazil nuts	High in omega-6 fats. Compared to other nuts these come out top for magnesium, are good for calcium and are a source of the antioxidant mineral selenium.
cashews	Good source of protein and folate, particularly good source of iron and zinc compared to other nuts and fibre-rich.
camellia tea oil	We may be introducing you to this fabulous oil but it is definitely worth seeking out. It has a very high smoke point making it an excellent choice for higher heat cooking in place of olive oil. Good source of vitamin E and other antioxidants.
linseeds (flaxseeds) and linseed oil	Linseeds are fairly unique in that they are one of the few plant sources rich in omega-3 fats. While not the long chain omega-3s found in fish and seafood, these shorter chain omega-3s are the next best thing. Linseed oil has a very low smoke point and therefore should never be used in cooking. Only use in salad dressings or over cereals. Delicious drizzled over Judy's porridge, page 147!
hazelnuts	Good source of protein and particularly rich in fibre compared to other nuts. Good source of many micronutrients including folate, iron and zinc.
nut spreads/butters	Rich in protein, fibre and numerous micronutrients. Excellent alternative to butter or margarine on your toast and highly nutritious for both adults and children (provided no allergies of course).
oily fish including Atlantic salmon, trout, silver perch, sardines, mackerel, herring and Queensland mullet	Provide the best source of the long chain omega-3 oils, eicosapentaenoic acid (EPA) and docosahexaenoic acid (DHA), essential to health. Also listed as a 5-star performer for protein (see pages 84 and 89-90).
olives and unrefined olive oil	A mainstay of the Mediterranean diet. Antioxidant-rich. Associated with low levels of heart disease. Great for salad dressings and as basic oil for cooking (but not high heat frying as oil will burn).
pecans	Not as much protein as other nuts but a good source of micronutrients including iron and zinc, fibre-rich and rich in antioxidants.
pine nuts	High in omega-6 fats. Particularly good for zinc compared to other nuts and good source of protein, fibre and a source of many micronutrients including folate and iron.
pistachios	Good source of protein and more than five times the vitamin A of other nuts. Good source of folate, iron and zinc.
seafood including oysters, mussels, squid, calamari, octopus	These foods are low in overall fat levels but we include them here as they do provide good levels of the long chain omega-3 oils (EPA and DHA) essential to health. Excellent sources of many micronutrients including iron and zinc. Also listed as a 5-star performer for protein (see pages 84 and 89).
sesame seeds and tahini (sesame butter)	High in omega-6 fats so watch total quantity to balance with omega-3s. Good source of iron, zinc, folate, protein and fibre. Tahini is particularly good for calcium.
sunflower seeds	High in omega-6 fats but you are likely to consume less than with the oil. Good source of iron, zinc, folate, protein, fibre and calcium.
walnuts	High in omega-6 fats. Good source of protein, fibre and a source of many of the micronutrients found in other nuts including folate, zinc and iron.

The table below summarises the attributes of each of our fat players including types of fat, key nutrients, processing factors and any additional information of note.

STAR PERFORMERS

Fat Source	Nutrient Summary
coconut and coconut oil	Coconuts have had a bad reputation, primarily as the fat present is highly saturated. However, these fats are not the same as those found in animal foods. The majority are medium chain triglycerides (MCTs) and do not raise cholesterol levels. In fact MCTs are readily burned as fuel leading many to suggest coconuts may assist weight control when used in place of other fats in the diet. Coconuts also possess anti-viral, anti-bacterial and anti-fungal properties and are used medicinally in many parts of the world. Many therefore consider coconuts a highly nutritious health food while others continue to be sceptical. We therefore reserve 5-star status until further research strengthens the evidence, but as a natural, minimally processed food that has been eaten for thousands of years we see it as a star performer.
macadamias	Don't quite make the 5-star performer category as, compared to other nuts, macadamias have less iron, zinc and other micronutrients, less protein and more total fat, saturated fat and kilojoules per serve. Nevertheless, they provide healthy fat and are a good source of fibre giving them star performer qualities.
peanuts, peanut butter and unrefined peanut oil	The predominant fat in peanuts is healthy monounsaturated fat. Peanuts and peanut butter are rich in fibre, a good source of B group vitamins, and a source of iron and zinc. However, peanuts don't make it to our 5-star performer category as they are heavily over-produced and over-processed by the food industry. This is of concern with the rising incidence of peanut allergies. There is also some concern that, because peanuts grow in the ground, in contrast to tree nuts, they absorb a far greater level of pesticides and other toxins. You can find organic peanuts and oil in good health food shops to eliminate this problem. Unrefined oil is not always easy to find as most is bulk produced and refined for high heat cooking. Otherwise, at least choose raw unsalted nuts and peanut butter with no added sugar or salt, and aim to broaden your taste to include other nuts.

GOOD PERFORMERS

Fat Source	Nutrient Summary
unrefined grapeseed oil	Main fat is polyunsaturated omega-6 fat so a good rather than star performer. This oil does have a high smoke point and can therefore be useful for high heat cooking.
unrefined sesame oil	Main fat is polyunsaturated omega-6 fat so a good rather than star performer. But imparts a delicious flavour in small quantities in stir-fries and salad dressings.
unrefined sunflower oil and safflower oil	Main fat is polyunsaturated omega-6 fat so a good rather than star performer, but is rich in the main fat-soluble antioxidant vitamin E.
whole-egg fresh mayonnaise	Look for one made with olive oil, whole eggs, vinegar and a simple ingredients list of only real foods with no preservatives, additives or other non-food items.

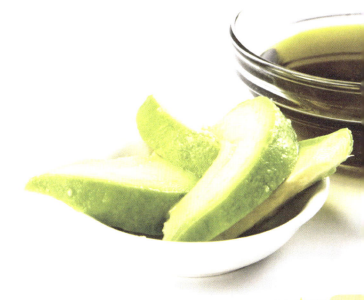

Player profiles – Fats (continued)

RESERVES

Fat Source	Nutrient Summary
butter	Butter fat is about 70 per cent saturated and therefore not a good fat to use regularly in your diet. However, butter does have some positive attributes. It is an excellent source of the fat-soluble vitamins A and D. It is also far less processed than margarines. When you really feel like a spread on some delicious bread or a special recipe calls for using butter, go ahead and enjoy—just don't make it a regular feature.
canola oil	We have our reservations about this oil. Not because of the numerous scare tactics employed by dubious websites; there is no evidence to support any of these claims (see page 115). But simply because it is manufactured to meet a demand for a stable healthy oil to be used by the food industry (olive oil is too expensive and cannot be used for all cooking applications). As such, it is refined and processed in order to be heat stable for cooking. However, it is predominantly healthy monounsaturated fat and as such it is not a bad choice for cooking. We simply cannot include it in the same star category as the many wonderful unrefined plant oils available.
corn oil	Main fat is polyunsaturated omega-6 fat and it is low in saturates. However, this is a highly processed, refined oil extracted using modern high-pressure techniques, with no real evidence of its long-term effect on health.
full-fat dairy products	A significant source of saturated fat in many people's diets and an easy one to cut down on; simply choose low-fat milks and yoghurts for everyday use. The exception is cheese—there are some good cheeses naturally lower in fat (check out page 113) but most manufactured low-fat cheese is also low on flavour. Go for the real thing but use sparingly. Full fat dairy foods do provide excellent levels of calcium and the fat-soluble vitamins A and D. Studies have also shown that cheese has a far smaller effect than butter on raising blood cholesterol. All up, a little of these foods will do no harm, but keep the emphasis on 'little'.
monounsaturated margarines, for example olive oil spread	Olive oil spread is not the same as olive oil, despite the pretty picture of an olive tree and Mediterranean scene on the box! While better than the polyunsaturated margarines since the major fat is the more neutral monounsaturated type, these are still highly processed products. If you love butter and find it hard to cut down, switching to one of these spreads is a move in the right direction, but far better to change how you eat to avoid needing a spread at all (see page 120).
plant sterol margarines	Plant sterols bind cholesterol in the gut, carrying it out the other end instead of being absorbed. Eat enough of it and there is no doubt that a plant sterol margarine can significantly reduce your blood cholesterol levels. If this then reduces the chances that you will need cholesterol-lowering medication then great. However, these are still processed margarines at the end of the day and as for all other margarines we cannot therefore recommend them as 5-star foods. A major problem with them is that you must eat enough of the margarine for it to have any effect. If you have high cholesterol, you may choose to give these margarines a shot. But we reckon you are far better changing your overall diet for long-term good health.
refined oils	High pressure and temperatures are used to extract the oil, which is then refined using solvents, traces of which remain in the oil. Bleaching and de-gumming are often further treatments used and both involve high temperature and/or chemicals. While there is no clear evidence that this is harmful unless trans fats are produced, some have questioned their safety. Spend a little more for a quality cold pressed oil.
rice bran oil	Gaining in popularity, this oil is extracted from the outer hull of rice grains. It contains a form of vitamin E that has been shown in some studies to lower cholesterol and be a powerful antioxidant. The fat profile is similar to peanut oil with the main fat being monounsaturated. However, the extraction method used involves high heat and chemical solvents therefore we question the healthfulness of the end product. It is certainly cheap but in the oil world price usually determines quality. The bottom line is this is a new oil without a track record of research.
roasted salted nuts including peanuts	While nuts and seeds are generally a healthy addition to your diet, they are not when they are roasted in oil and heavily coated with salt. For healthy blood pressure we need more potassium and less sodium (salt).
soy bean oil	Main fat is polyunsaturated omega-6 fat and it is low in saturates. But not an oil with a long history of use and can only be produced using modern high-pressure extraction techniques. Widely used by the food industry and often hydrogenated for use in margarines and other food products—avoid these products.

Note: In our overall diet, we want to ensure we don't allow the polyunsaturated omega-6 fats to dominate over the omega-3s. A balance of the two fat types is crucial. Oils are the pure fat extracted from the nut or seed and are therefore a far more significant source of the fat than eating the whole food. For this reason we don't include

LIABILITIES

Fat Source	Nutrient Summary
commercially baked products including doughnuts, cakes, pastries and biscuits	Let's face it, most of us love a sweet treat and we certainly don't mean to banish your favourites to the 'never' category. You can have your cake and eat it, so long as you choose the right cake. Commercially produced products are likely to use the cheapest ingredients and that means the cheapest, least nutritious fats. These products are high in saturated fat, can also have significant levels of trans fat, and are energy-dense and nutrient-poor. See pages 136-7 for delicious and nutritious sweet treats to opt for instead.
commercially deep-fried food and fast food	A major source of the worst kind of fat—trans fat. Caused by repeatedly heating oils to a high temperature which changes the physical structure of the fat. These products tend to be high in total fat, energy-dense but nutrient-poor. Need we say more?
commercial mayonnaise	Read the ingredients list to see whether it seems a healthy choice or not. Commercial mayonnaise has preservatives, additives and flavourings added and is usually based on processed egg substitute and undesirable oils. A far better choice is a fresh mayonnaise found in the refrigerated section that lists only real food ingredients … even better to make your own using olive oil and omega-3-rich free range eggs.
lard	You can still get lard in the supermarket so someone is still buying it. Don't! This is pure animal fat (100 per cent fat compared to 80 per cent fat in butter). It is extremely high in saturated fat and cholesterol, and doesn't even provide good quantities of fat-soluble vitamins as butter does. We will concede, however, that lard is preferable to using a heavily processed and refined plant fat for use in pastry making and certain other cooking applications—in these instances occasional consumption will not harm you.
low- and reduced-fat spreads	It might surprise you that we think these are dreadful and most people assume this is a healthy choice. However, these are highly processed, manufactured products that give you a false sense of security. Research has shown that we tend to use more spread if told it is low-fat, than if told it is the full-fat original product. The ingredient list should be enough to put you off. Skip it and instead use good quality healthy fats in moderation.
palm oil	This fat is often assumed to be healthy being a plant fat, and may be labelled as simply vegetable fat. However, it is one of the few plant fats to be extremely high in saturated fat. This makes it a stable fat and therefore often favoured in food production. Look for it in ingredient lists of pre-prepared and packaged foods and if the oil is simply listed as vegetable oil assume it is palm oil and avoid.
polyunsaturated margarines	These are usually based on sunflower or safflower oil and are marketed as a healthy choice. However, as with low-fat spreads, these are highly processed products and, let's face it, sunflower margarine is not the same as sunflower oil and a far cry from eating the whole sunflower seed.
salad dressing (cream)	As with commercial mayonnaise, read the ingredient list for reasons not to consume this food product. Making your own delicious and nutritious salad dressing is neither difficult nor time-consuming when you know how.
shortening	Sometimes this is made from animal fat, but more usually it is hydrogenated vegetable fat. As such it contains the worst kind of fat—trans fat. Certainly avoid using it yourself but you are more likely to be unwittingly consuming it in processed, packaged foods.
stick/block margarines	Not so common in Australia but widely used in the US and elsewhere. These are more solid margarines used as a cheap alternative to butter. The problem is oil is liquid at room temperature. Therefore to make a solid product the oil has to be structurally changed to be more similar to saturated fat (think of fluid olive oil compared to hard butter). The result is the significant production of trans fats. We can think of no reason to ever use these products.
suet and tallow	Suet is raw beef or mutton fat and tallow is made from suet. Both are highly saturated fat. While you may not ever think you consume these fats, they are used in many foods such as Christmas pudding, mincemeat pies and many pastry goods. Vegetable suet is made from palm oil and is therefore not much better.
visible meat fat	The white solid fat you can see on meat, under the skin on poultry, in salami and sausages, pork crackling and marbled through many meats is a major source of unhealthy saturated fat and cholesterol. Remove it where you can and choose lean cuts of meat without marbling.

omega-6-rich oils in our fabulous choices as a better choice is a neutral monounsaturated fat or oil that provides omega-3s. However, nuts and seeds that contain omega-6s have other nutritional attributes and the total amount of fat you get from eating the whole food is far less, therefore most of these are included as 5-star choices.

Chapter 6

Drinks

Drinks often get forgotten when it comes to making diet and lifestyle changes in the name of good health. In fact the only common message we tend to hear is that we need to drink more water. This is certainly true for many, but given the vast array of drinks now on offer we really need to know more.

One of the problems with drinks is that they are very easily absorbed giving us ready access to the kilojoules they contain. This might sound a good thing but, since most of us are watching our waistlines if not actively trying to reduce them, these easily absorbed kilojoules are not of such a great quality. Furthermore, drinks by-pass many of the appetite feedback systems to the brain that happen when we eat solid foods. In short, this means it is all too easy to knock back hundreds of extra kilojoules without your body reducing your appetite and switching off your rumbling tummy. The result—you eat the same but add all those extra kilojoules and wonder why you are gaining weight or failing to lose it.

But it's not all down to kilojoules—there are many nutrients and phytochemicals to be found in the drinks we choose that can do us much benefit beyond providing simple hydration. Teas and vegetable juices are great examples. On the downside, drinks can be kilojoule-free yet be loaded with undesirable additives, flavourings and sweeteners that have the potential to do much harm over the long term. So, let's look beyond water and consider the other drinks that may be frequent tipples or tempt us with confusing advertising and image.

Rolling out the drinks players

Each player was assigned a division based on its nutritional profile. The criteria for the selection process were based on their ability to hydrate the body without negatively influencing its performance. Consideration was given to energy density, antioxidants/phytochemicals, nutrients supplied, sugar and sweeteners added, and other processing factors.

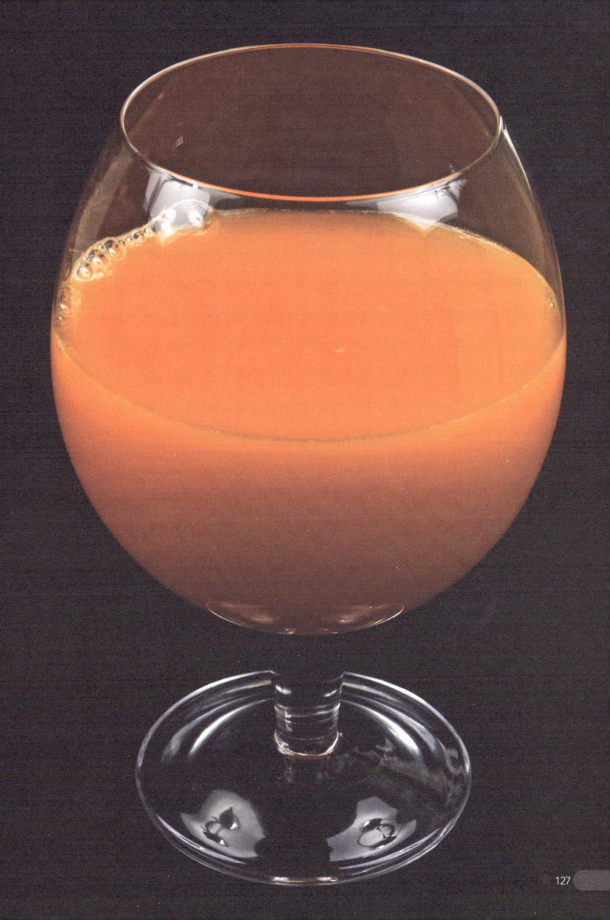

Ranking the Players/Player Profiles – Drinks

5-STAR PERFORMERS

Drink	Nutrient Summary
fresh vegetable juice	Low energy density and packed with nutrients. A good way to boost your veggie intake. Juice for yourself or buy one with no undesirable additives.
herbal teas	Most are kilojoule-free. Herbal teas are a caffeine-free alternative to coffee and tea. Some have mild therapeutic benefits, such as chamomile to aid sleep. However, in excess, some can discolour the enamel of your teeth.
rooibos tea	Another energy and caffeine-free drink. Rooibos is a red leaf tea from South Africa. Rich in antioxidants. It can be drunk with or without milk and makes a good caffeine-free alternative to tea.
sparkling or still mineral water	Again it's kilojoule-free and provides small quantities of minerals. The bubbles can make a refreshing change and can help if you're trying to cut back on soft drinks or reduce alcohol intake at night.
tea—black, green, white and oolong	All these teas are a rich source of antioxidants and tea drinking is associated with lower risk of heart disease and several cancers including stomach, oesophageal, skin and ovarian cancer. Green tea is not to everyone's taste and can make some people slightly nauseous. Take heart that, despite this tea's good publicity, all tea promotes good health with no one coming out on top to date. Do be aware that all tea, including green, contains caffeine (less than half the amount found in coffee), but the caffeine intake from drinking four to five cups of tea a day is not associated with any harmful effect. Tea does also contain tannins that inhibit the absorption of plant-based iron. Avoid this problem by drinking your tea between, and not with, your meals.
water	Kilojoule-free and quite simply the best and cheapest way to hydrate the body. No distinction made here between tap, filtered and bottled water—bottled water is not necessarily better for your health. Tap water can, in some parts of the country, taste unpleasant. If that's the case where you live buy bottled or invest in a filter.

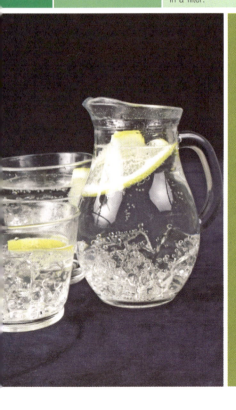

STAR PERFORMERS

Drink	Nutrient Summary
fresh vegetable and fruit juice	With the added fruit the energy density increases but it is still a nutrient-rich drink and the addition of fruit makes it more palatable for most people. Make sure the ratio of vegetables to fruit is more than 2:1 using fruit to slightly sweeten only.
natural cocoa powder (not to be confused with drinking chocolate powder—this has far less cocoa, added sugar and often additional flavourings/additives)	The native Kuna Indians of Panama drink three to four cups of homemade cocoa a day and have very low rates of high blood pressure and heart disease. Researchers have attributed this to the high flavonoid antioxidants in cocoa. Natural cocoa powder is the least processed form of chocolate and as such it retains far higher levels of these antioxidants. Plus it has no fat and no added sugar. Try adding a teaspoon to warm skim milk for a healthy chocolate fix. However, cocoa does contain small amounts of caffeine and much higher levels of a similar compound called theobromine—this has similar, but far milder, effects on the central nervous system as caffeine. However, you are extremely unlikely to eat enough cocoa powder for this to be a problem!
soda water	This is just carbonated water but it is higher in sodium (salt) than most other waters. Nevertheless it provides kilojoule-free hydration.

The table below summarises the attributes of each of our drinks players including energy density, nutrients present, processing factors and any additional information of note.

GOOD PERFORMERS

Drink	Nutrient Summary
alcohol including wine, spirits and beer	Wine has had all the good press but, in fact, all alcoholic drinks, when consumed in small amounts regularly, are good for the heart and circulatory system and probably reduce the risk of type 2 diabetes and gallstones. It's true that red wine contains more antioxidants than other drinks and these may be of benefit; but let's be honest, these can be found elsewhere. Don't fool yourself into thinking a bottle of red a night is good for you! In excess, alcohol is incredibly harmful, damaging your liver, your heart, increasing your risk of breast cancer, accidents and depression, while clouding your judgment and affecting what you choose to eat. By all means enjoy a couple of drinks a day, but give yourself at least two alcohol-free days a week.
coffee	There are many potential health benefits from coffee (see pages 132-3). For example, it improves alertness, concentration and brain performance, exercise performance and may assist weight control by encouraging fat 'burning' and boosting metabolism. It also stimulates bowel movement, a welcome relief for many. Like tea, coffee contains a high level of antioxidants, but unlike tea there is no solid evidence that coffee consumption reduces the risk of heart disease and cancer (but neither is there evidence to suggest coffee increases your risk). Coffee (and caffeine) consumption has been shown to lower the risk of Parkinson's disease and diabetes. However, it has more than double the caffeine content of tea and in excess this can overly stimulate the central nervous system resulting in restlessness, insomnia, anxiety and tremors. Others find coffee irritates the gut and may make conditions such as heartburn worse. Drinking more than four cups of coffee a day may increase your risk of osteoporosis. Finally, be discerning about what you put in your coffee—full-fat milk or cream, sugars and flavoured syrups can result in a kilojoule-packed drink. Stick to a maximum of three a day, use skim milk if you like it white and don't add sugar.
decaffeinated coffee using the Swiss water® process	This method uses only water to remove the caffeine and is therefore completely chemical free, unlike most other decaf coffees. For information on where you can buy it in Australia (and worldwide) visit **www.swisswater.com**. Of course the removal of the caffeine may also remove some of the benefits of regular coffee. Note: If you suffer from heartburn, studies have shown no difference between decaf and regular coffee, suggesting that it is not the caffeine to blame.
fresh fruit juice	A nutrient-rich drink that is healthy in small amounts. But many nutrients are lost from the whole fruit, especially fibre. Significant source of extra kilojoules since it is relatively energy-dense and serving sizes can be enormous making it very easy to over-consume. Better to eat the whole fruit instead. Enjoy the occasional fresh juice when you are out, but don't keep in the fridge at home.
low-fat fruit smoothies made with fruit, low-fat milk and yoghurt with no additives	Smoothies can be a healthy, satisfying and filling snack or meal, provided they are made with the right ingredients. Use low-fat milk and yoghurt combined with fresh or frozen fruit. The combination is low GI and can be helpful in keeping you full until the next meal. Good breakfast option for those who don't like solid food first thing. Be wary of the enormous serving sizes, added cream or ice cream and various undesirable additives that can be found in commercial smoothies.
skim milk	All the calcium and protein of whole milk with none of the fat. The protein in milk is also rich in the amino acid leucine, which is thought to assist in preserving muscle (and therefore increasing fat loss) during weight loss, and promoting growth and repair of muscles after exercise. The combination of calcium and leucine may be particularly beneficial during weight loss although this has yet to be substantiated. Also has a low GI and can help keep hunger at bay between meals. A warm cup of milk before bed can help you to fall asleep. However, milk is not suitable for those with lactose intolerance and there is some concern that high intakes may increase the risk of ovarian and prostate cancers. Until this is resolved we cannot yet be confident about the safety of a high intake of milk. Stick to one to two cups a day to gain the benefits while limiting any potential risk.

Ranking the Player/Player Profiles – Drinks (continued)

RESERVES

Drink	Nutrient Summary
chemically decaffeinated coffee	Most decaf coffee is made using beans that have had the caffeine removed using chemical solvents. There is inevitably residue of the chemicals present (albeit in small quantities) but whether this has any effect on health is not known. However, one US study found that decaf, and not regular coffee, increased heart disease risk. The reason is not known and one study is not definitive proof. Nevertheless it cautions us not to make the assumption that decaf must be healthier.
flavoured milk	Contains a lot of sugar and/or artificial sweeteners and many contain additional artificial flavourings and other additives. They are also usually bought in large sizes—the label will say it contains two or more serves but who only drinks half the bottle?! They are, however, low GI and OK for an occasional filling snack when you are on the run. For a healthier choice, choose one that is made with low-fat milk, advertises a lower sugar content and read the ingredients list to ensure no other additives.
flavoured water	Marketed as healthy but these are just water with added sugar and flavourings. Certainly they have less sugar and kilojoules than soft drinks but much better to make your own with sparkling water and a splash of fruit juice.
fruit and vegetable juices with added preservatives and colour	Read the label—many seemingly 'fresh' fruit and vegetable juices have undesirable additives.
hot chocolate	Although some goodness in the cocoa, drinking chocolate has a lot of sugar added and sometimes artificial flavours, preservatives and other additives too. Read the label. Café hot chocolate can also be loaded with dairy fat with the addition of cream and/or whole milk. They also tend to use a lot of drinking chocolate powder. Ask for skim milk and less powder.

LIABILITIES

Drink	Nutrient Summary
alcoholic pop drinks	Sometimes called 'chicky' drinks, these are a dreadful combination of too much sugar, alcohol, flavourings, colourings and other additives. They are too easy to drink quickly and to drink too many of them. Have a glass of wine and a second with sparkling water instead.
cordial	Extremely high in sugar and often with added artificial colours, flavours and preservatives. Don't drink it yourself and definitely don't buy it for the kids.
diet soft drinks	Sorry we are just not fans. They might be almost kilojoule free, but they use artificial sweeteners, colours, and flavourings, and they still damage your teeth by eroding the enamel. If you need to lose weight they are a step in the right direction from regular soft drinks, but quickly move on and get into the water habit instead!
energy drinks	These might sound a good idea when you need a lift, but these are just soft drinks with added caffeine—and usually lots of it. Be aware that guarana might be all 'natural' but it is just more caffeine. The kilojoule content is often even higher than regular soft drinks.
flavoured coffee syrups	This is just lots of refined sugar usually with artificial flavours, colours and other undesirable additives.
soft drinks/sodas	Full of sugar, soft drinks provide an all too easy to over-consume package of kilojoules. As such they have a major role to play in our escalating weight problem. They are also incredibly bad for your teeth, promoting both decay and erosion. Just don't drink them.

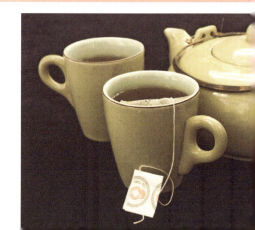

Tea

Tea is the most commonly consumed beverage in the world after water. Its origins are in China where tea has been enjoyed for more than 4000 years. White, green, black and oolong tea all come from the same camellia plant, but undergo different processing to give them their characteristic flavours.

Essentially, the difference between green and black tea is that green tea undergoes less processing, it is simply the steamed and dried leaves of the plant. Whereas, to make black tea, the leaves undergo an additional stage of oxidation before drying. This produces a darker, generally stronger colour and flavour. White tea is a specialty of the Chinese province Fujian and is made from less mature leaves than green tea, and is the least processed tea. Oolong tea is a traditional Chinese tea and is somewhere in between black and green tea being semi-oxidised. If you don't like the slightly grassy taste of green tea, oolong may be for you.

All teas contain the potent antioxidants collectively called polyphenols. However, the level of processing affects the type of polyphenol present. White and green teas have a far higher quantity of catechins, shown in human and animal studies to have the potential to reduce the risk of heart disease and cancer. Green tea in particular has received a lot of positive press regarding its health benefits, some of which has been attributed to the catechin EGCG (epigallocatechin gallate) found in abundance in these less processed teas. However, other studies have found no difference in total antioxidant capacity of different teas, including directly comparing green and black tea. It's just that the oxidation of the leaves to make black tea produces a different polyphenol group called theaflavins. Whether there are greater benefits to health of one or other of these antioxidants is not really known. In fact, to say one tea is healthier than another seems to us to be splitting hairs. There is convincing evidence for the benefits of both green and black tea, the most commonly consumed, and so which one you choose to drink is up to you. Why not stock your pantry with different types to be sure of the full range of tea antioxidants?

Do be aware, however, that black, green, white and oolong teas all contain caffeine. This is considerably less than coffee and the caffeine from four to five cups of tea a day has not been shown to cause any harmful effects, while potentially providing great benefit. Nevertheless, if you are sensitive to the effects of caffeine, or are pregnant or breastfeeding, moderate your tea consumption accordingly. The only other negative of tea drinking is that the tannins in tea reduce the absorption of plant-based iron. That's a simple one to solve—drink your tea between and not with your meals. This is particularly important for vegetarians and vegans. The question of whether adding milk to your tea affects the nutritional benefits is not really known, but the weight of evidence so far suggests not. We recommend you stick to a splash of skim milk if you so wish, but skip the sugar.

If you want a tea that is caffeine-free, you can choose form herbal teas or rooibos. These are not technically teas, and should more correctly be called tisanes. Herbal teas are simply infusions made with herbs, flowers, fruit, roots, spices or other parts of the plant. They do not therefore contain the same polyphenols as tea, nor confer the same health benefits. Also be aware that many of the health claims made on the packets of herbal teas are not proven and are dubious at best. Nevertheless, they are caffeine-free, kilojoule-free and may have other healthful qualities such as promoting relaxation and aiding sleep. Rooibos comes from South Africa and is becoming increasingly popular here. It does boast a high content of antioxidants and is both caffeine- and tannin-free. You make it in the same way as black tea, but may want to leave it to brew a little longer to allow the full flavour to develop. In South Africa they usually add milk and sugar, but it is delicious without and is of course completely kilojoule-free when enjoyed in this way.

Coffee

Coffee has been enjoyed for several hundred years and seems to have always divided opinion on whether or not it is good for us. Coffee has a mild stimulatory effect on the central nervous system, attributed almost entirely to the presence of caffeine. This tends to wake you up and make you feel more alert. But does it do us any harm? The evidence is not nearly as damning as you might think and in fact coffee may even be doing us some good.

Caffeine can certainly make you anxious, but only at doses above about 600 mg of caffeine (Liebermann, 1992). Since a typical cup of coffee contains 80–140 mg of caffeine, that equates to consuming several cups. Normal intakes of caffeine, equivalent to two to three cups of coffee a day, have not been shown to increase anxiety in either healthy subjects or those with existing anxiety disorders. There is even some evidence to show that small amounts of caffeine can reduce anxiety. Caffeine has also been shown to increase several aspects of mental performance, including the ability to process new stimuli and increase the amount of information processed. So a coffee before that all-important presentation may well help to calm your nerves and improve your performance. There may even be a longer-term benefit. One study measured the cognitive function of over 1500 elderly men and women using 12 standard tests (Johnson-Kozlow et al, 2002). They found that the women with higher lifetime coffee consumption performed better in six of these tests.

Coffee may benefit the brain in other ways too. Two studies—one retrospective case-control study (Maia & de Mendonca, 2002) and the other a prospective study involving more than 1500 Canadians (Lindsay, 2002)—have shown an inverse relationship between coffee consumption and Alzheimer's disease. Definitive conclusions cannot be drawn from only two studies but these results have prompted further research. There is stronger evidence for a link with Parkinson's disease. A recent meta-analysis of 13 studies to meet the inclusion criteria, demonstrated a 31 per cent reduction in risk of developing Parkinson's in those who drank coffee compared to those who did not (Hernán et al, 2002). This reduction in risk was even greater among men and the relationship was linear meaning that the more coffee they drank the lower their risk became. In women, the picture was complicated by whether or not hormone replacement therapy was used post-menopause. Consumption of coffee lowered the risk of Parkinson's in women who did not use HRT, but raised the risk in those who did. This suggests there may be some interaction between a component of coffee and exogenous oestrogen use, but we need more research before firm conclusions can be made. Nevertheless, taken together these results tell a promising story for the benefits of coffee on the short- and long-term functioning of the brain.

Without doubt caffeine can affect sleep—both the time it takes you to fall asleep and the duration of sleep. But we are not all affected to the same degree. While some can drink coffee at bedtime without adverse effect, others find a coffee at breakfast causes them to be tossing and turning that night. This can partly be explained by habituation—the more coffee you drink, the less it affects you—but undoubtedly we all have an individual sensitivity to caffeine. For the majority avoiding caffeine in the evening will prevent any unwanted effect on sleep.

Coffee has been shown to be of benefit in the treatment of asthma, probably by acting as a bronchodilator. As far back as the late 1800s there are reports of caffeine being used to assist breathing in asthmatics. More recently, two-large scale population studies—one in Italy (Pagano et al, 1988) and the other in the US (Schwartz & Weiss, 1992)—have found the risk of asthma to be almost 30 per cent lower in coffee drinkers compared to non-coffee drinkers.

Much is made of the antioxidant content of tea, but coffee has in fact been shown to have a greater total antioxidant power than other beverages including green or black tea, herbal tea or cocoa! The types of antioxidants present are of course different in each and it remains to be seen whether the characteristics of coffee really do prove to be protective. Epidemiological studies have failed to come to definitive conclusions about associations between coffee consumption and cardiovascular disease. In part this has been due to confounding where coffee drinking acts as a marker for some other lifestyle factor that is known to increase risk. Several studies have found that coffee increases blood levels of homocysteine. However, current opinion is divided as to whether homocysteine levels are in fact a risk factor. Either way, since the effect of coffee is relatively minor it seems unlikely that there is any real effect on risk of the cardiovascular disease. As far as coffee consumption and cancer goes, there have been numerous case-control and cohort studies to look for an association. A 2000 review concluded that there was no evidence to suggest a link between moderate coffee consumption and cancer of any site (Tavani & La Vecchia, 2000). It seems clear that for both cardiovascular disease and cancer prevention there are far more important dietary changes you can make.

The other big chronic disease affecting Australians is type 2 diabetes and there may be good news for coffee lovers here. The famous Nurses Health Study in the US reported early in 2006 that moderate consumption of both coffee and decaffeinated coffee may lower the risk of type 2 diabetes in younger and middle-aged women (van Dam et al, 2006). Caffeine could clearly not explain the effect and so researchers are now looking at other constituents of coffee for possible answers. A second study published the same year showed positive effects of coffee on several markers of glucose metabolism (Bidel et al, 2006). Coffee consumption was linked to lower blood glucose levels, both in the fasting and postprandial state, and lower insulin levels. Over time this could explain how coffee lowers diabetes risk. However, not all studies agree and much more research is needed to draw firm conclusions.

You might think that the effects of coffee on the gut are unquestionable. But even here there is conflicting evidence. There is certainly evidence that coffee can exacerbate heartburn in some people, although not all. If you suffer regularly you could try switching to decaf as that seems to help some—but, again, the published research gives conflicting results. Since decaf affects some just as much as regular coffee it seems likely that some other constituent of coffee is to blame. There is no evidence that coffee increases the risk of stomach ulcers or causes indigestion.

In conclusion the potential hazards of coffee means that we cannot class it as a 5-star drink choice, but the rarely talked about positives of this traditional drink really do make its bad reputation unjust. We have therefore listed coffee, perhaps rather controversially, as a good performer. Just exercise moderation over how much you drink. More to the point is the way you drink it. The American-style coffee bars with oversize cups, a vast range of syrupy, artificially flavoured additives and enormous quantities of milk and/or cream added, can turn a relatively healthy, kilojoule free drink into a nutritional nightmare. Keep it simple—skip the extras and choose skim milk.

Chapter 7

Treats

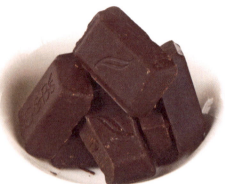

Although at the top of the food pyramid model, and therefore should be a small part of a healthy diet, treats are nevertheless an important part. The pleasure of eating and the sensory experience of consuming certain foods has always been an essential part of our relationship with food. The saddest thing we have ever heard in relation to food is a fitness instructor at one of our seminars in Sydney saying they would much prefer to take a pill to provide all the nutrition they need rather than have to eat real food. Let's hope we never, ever get to that point! Look at any culture or community around the world and food is a part of celebration, socialising, commiseration, mourning—in fact almost every human event you can think of. Treats play a part in this and keep our relationship with food a healthy one. Guilt and eating have no business together—if you respect your body and enjoy your food then treats, whatever they may be, can healthily and happily be consumed. The key is all in the quantity and quality of *all* foods in your diet.

Nevertheless, not all treats are equal with some providing positive nutritional aspects and only a little potential damage, while others have nothing nutritional to offer (other than kilojoules) and much that can do harm. You can afford to indulge more often in the former without compromising your health and wellbeing. To that end we hope to guide you by relegating popular treats to the appropriate division. You'll notice there are no 5-star performers here as no treat is completely devoid of potential harm, but there are several star performers that we can recommend. Enjoy!

Rolling out the treat players

Each player in the table on page 136-138 was assigned a division based on its nutritional profile. The criteria for the selection process were based on their ability to provide pleasure without doing too much damage. Consideration was given to the energy density, type of fat, processing factors and the quantity of sugar & /or salt added.

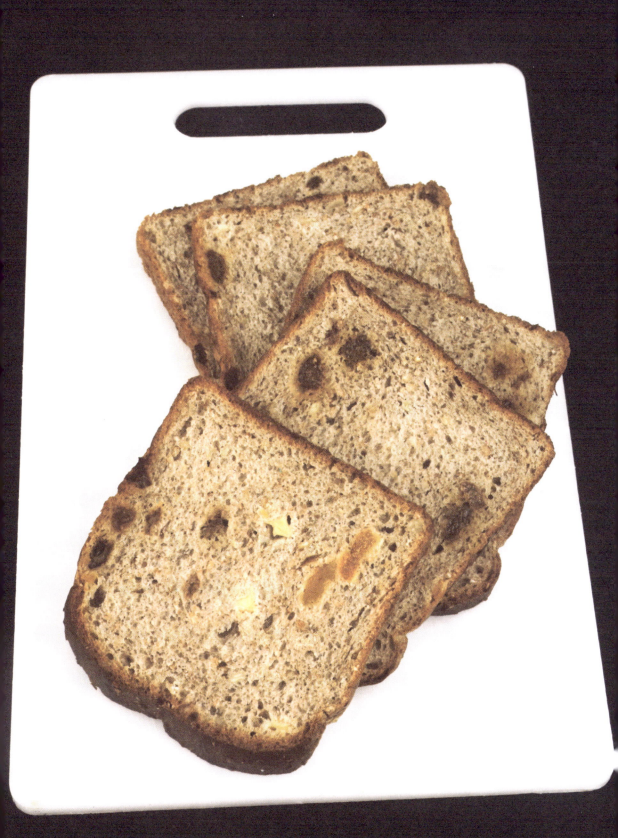

Ranking the Players/Player Profiles – Treats

STAR PERFORMERS

Treat	Key Points
dark chocolate (min. 70 per cent cocoa)	The cocoa in chocolate is a rich source of flavonoid antioxidants that are thought to be beneficial to health. They may be cardioprotective by preventing the damage to LDL-cholesterol that results in atherosclerosis, and may also lower blood pressure. Dark chocolate contains the most cocoa and therefore the highest level of antioxidants. There is little difference in fat or kilojoules between dark, milk and white chocolate, but the strong, slightly bitter flavour of dark chocolate tends to satisfy you and put a brake on how much you eat. Although high in saturated fat, the type found in cocoa butter does not raise cholesterol. (The same may not be true for lower quality chocolate made with cheaper fats.) This is still an energy-dense food nonetheless so exercise quality over quantity.
fruit bread	Dense fruit bread made with wholemeal flour and lots of fruit has a low GI (not so for many commercial sliced raisin toast varieties). In addition, the dried fruit provides many nutrients (covered in our fruit section). Delicious served with low-fat ricotta. Read the labels of commercial varieties—many have undesirable additives including preservatives—and look for one with a simple list of all food ingredients.
100 per cent fruit bars/roll ups	Although they're not a good as fresh fruit, these treats are a handy no-mess addition to the school lunchbox. With many of the nutrients of fresh fruit retained, they're easy to transport and provide a great source of energy. Make sure you check the labels before purchase—not all are 100 per cent fruit and some have added sugar, flavours, colours and other artificial additives. This also affects the GI. While those made with 100 per cent fruit have so far come out low, those with 65 per cent fruit or less can have extremely high GI values.
wholemeal fruit-filled bars/biscuits	A higher fibre snack than most sweet biscuits and lower in refined sugar. Search the GI database for those with a low GI for the best choice (www.glycemicindex.com).
mixed dried fruit with raw nuts and seeds (trail mix)	A good high-fibre, low-GI snack but is far more energy-dense than fresh fruit. Enjoy in moderation. Drying fruit is essentially a great way to preserve fresh fruit and give it a conveniently long shelf life. Most nutrients are preserved with the exception of vitamin C. Sulphur dioxide is usually added to commercial dried fruits to preserve a bright colour. You can avoid this additive by choosing organic sun-dried fruit—it will be darker in colour but the flavour is usually also better. Adding raw nuts and seeds adds fibre, protein and healthy fats for a more balanced, filling snack.
roasted unsalted nuts	Roasted nuts may become rancid if they've been stored for too long. Provided you buy them from a store with a quick turnover they make a good snack. They do have a high energy density so be careful not to overeat. A standard serve is around 30 grams, the equivalent to approximately 30 almonds, 10 brazil nuts and 20 cashews.
homemade oat/muesli bars	Made with raw muesli and a small amount of butter and sugar, homemade muesli bars make a good high fibre snack with all the nutrients found in muesli.

GOOD PERFORMERS

Treat	Key Points
air-popped corn	Cooked without fat and no added sugar, pop corn is a good high-fibre, low-energy snack. It does have a high GI so don't expect it to fill you up. Best avoided if you're managing high blood sugar.
biscotti	Traditional biscotti contains no oil or butter and is therefore a low-fat treat. They are made with white flour and sugar but the almonds help to reduce their GI and boost the overall nutritional value. Many hybrid recipes add chocolate chunks, cocoa powder etc. and are not as good as plain biscotti.
banana bread (un-iced)	Largely dependent on the recipe and the type of flour, fat and quantity of sugar used, some nutrients from the banana make this treat better than many others.
carrot cake (un-iced)	Largely dependent on the recipe and the type of flour, fat and quantity of sugar used, some nutrients from the carrot make this treat better than many others.
bhuja mix	Known also as Bombay mix, this snack is made from high-fibre lentils, nuts, chickpea chips, sultanas and spices. The downside is it's deep-fried!
bran and fruit muffins	Another treat that is largely dependent on the recipe (and SIZE!). Select muffins made with part wholemeal flour, fruit and bran that are no bigger than 7 centimetres in diameter. They make a reasonable high-fibre snack.
friands	The almond meal and egg whites add some nutritional value to these cakes. The small size also makes them easier to enjoy without overeating.
fruit cake	A dense fruit cake is a high energy snack, but offers a number of nutrients and fibre from the fruit.

The table below summarises the attributes of each of our treat players including energy density, any health benefits, fats present, processing factors and other additional information of note.

GOOD PERFORMERS

Treat	Key Points
homemade fruit pies and crumbles	Made from naturally sweet fruit with little added sugar and a pastry or crumble top these are not too bad.
chocolate-coated nuts and raisins	The health benefits of the nuts and raisins are offset by the low-quality, high-sugar/high-fat chocolate coating.
milk chocolate	Higher in fat and sugar than dark chocolate but still contains some of the health benefits from the cocoa.
wheaten/oat biscuits	Some fibre from the wheat and oats.
real liquorice	Liquorice comes from the root of a shrub approximately 50 times sweeter than sugar. The confectionery is made from molasses with small quantities of liquorice and anise. Molasses is a thick syrup by-product produced during the production of table sugar. It does contain small amounts of several nutrients including iron, magnesium, vitamin K and potassium, but it is still primarily extracted sugar so don't be fooled into thinking it is a health product. When buying liquorice, check the ingredients to ensure it's made from molasses as cheaper versions are simply artificially flavoured confectionery and not the real thing. A serve of liquorice should be no greater than one 10 centimetre piece.
salted/tamari roasted nuts	A good source of fibre and other nutrients from nuts, but easy to overeat. High in energy and salt.

RESERVES

Treat	Key Points
commercial fruit pies	Commercially bought pies are often loaded in sugar. With both a base and lid, they are high in energy and some are made with damaging trans fats.
muffins	Made from white processed flour, sugar and generally oversized. High GI.
Anzac biscuits	High in fat and sugar.
boxed chocolates	Candy and toffee fillings are full of sugar, and many other commercial additives.
caramelised nuts	Very high in refined sugar and not great for your teeth.
scones	High GI, made with white bleached flour and fat.
white chocolate	Made from fat and sugar with no cocoa.
chocolate-coated biscuits	Poor quality chocolate, and high in fat and sugar with added colourings make these a poor choice.
muesli bars	Generally thought as healthy, they are very high in sugar (from glucose) and high in fat. A very high energy food.
pancakes	High GI, made with white bleached flour and fat. Premixed commercial pancake products have extra additives and are even worse.
uniced sponge cakes and cup cakes	High GI bleached white flour, butter and sugar form the basis of all sponges.
pretzels	Marketed as a healthier snack, they have an exceptionally high GI, and are high in salt.
soy chips	Considered healthy, soy chips are deep-fried, high in salt and energy.
salted chips	High in salt and energy—like all salted products, easy to overeat.
homemade or quality ice-cream	Made from thickened cream and sugar—natural ingredients and therefore a far better choice than those loaded with artificial additives and flavours. However high in saturated fat and significant kilojoules so not an everyday food.

Treats

Ranking the Players/Player Profiles – Treats (continued)

LIABILITIES

Treat	Key Points
boiled sweets	Boiled sugar, water, artificial colouring and flavours. At best they work on rotting the teeth.
jelly and jellied confectionery	Sugar, artificial colouring and additives.
iced sponges, cupcakes and cream cakes	High GI bleached white flour, butter and sugar form the basis of all sponges. Cream and icing lift the fat and sugar content making them worse, and adding colouring to the icing worse again.
chocolate cakes and brownies	Loaded in fat and sugar these are very high in energy.
chocolate-coated toffee	Very high in kilojoules and refined sugar. The stickiness makes these treats a disaster for teeth.
commercial icecream including choc tops and ice-cream confectionery	Made from poor quality vegetable fat and sugar, usually with added artificial flavourings and colouring. Lots of kilojoules for very few nutrients.
cheese cake	High in saturated fat and kilojoules.
nougat	Boiled sugar, with colouring and a few nuts.
sausage rolls	Very high in saturated fat and likely to contain trans fats in the pastry.
Chiko rolls	Deep fried battered sausage—high in saturated fat and loaded with kilojoules. Also likely to contain trans fats.
party pies	Energy-dense and a source of trans and saturated fats.
protein bars	Marketed as healthy but why should processed protein be any better for us than processed anything else?! In addition they are often full of artificial additives and flavourings.
flavoured chips and snack biscuits	High concentration of salt and artificial flavourings. Energy-dense and full of the wrong types of fat.
sweet pastries	High GI, loaded with kilojoules and the wrong types of fat.
creamy desserts	Energy-dense and high in saturated fat, cholesterol and sugar.
doughnuts	Deep-fried, white processed flour and lots of sugar. Iced doughnuts are even worse.
pancake and cake mixes	Extra additives added to preserve the main ingredients.

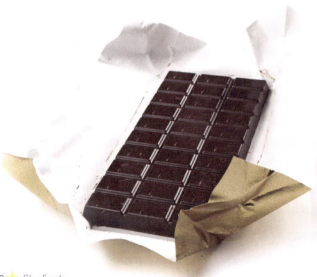

Chapter 8

What's Wrong with Most Diets?

Given what you know now, from the information on each food group, you can see when the hierarchy of our 5-Star Performers through to the Liabiltities, is applied to various popular diets, and plotted onto a food pyramid, they fail to give you everything you need and, overall, compromise your health.

In this typical diet illustrated in Figure 8.1, which has contributed to producing the fattest generation of all time, you can see from our pyramid that while there is a relatively good intake of vegetables (with perhaps a few no-fat high-GI baked potatoes in there), there are far too many bad choices of carbohydrates and insufficient proteins. Low-fat biscuits, cakes and other high-energy, high-GI carbohydrates fill the cupboards, and our stomachs. And, worst of all, many treats that we consider to be 'liabilities' since they have no nutritional value whatsoever are considered OK.

The high-protein dieter following the plan shown in Figure 8.2 may lose weight quickly—but at what cost? High in 'liability' fats, little thought given to the quality of the proteins, and not nearly enough vegetables or fruit are all likely to increase the risk of chronic disease such as heart disease and cancers. The lack of quality carbohydrates makes exercise difficult, and since these provide the best source of glucose to feed the brain, concentration and mental task performance are impaired.

The lack of fibre means that constipation is a common problem and bowel health is seriously compromised. Furthermore, if you manage to get the carbs low enough to force your body into what is known as a ketogenic state, your breath will smell and your head will ache. Yes, you will be burning fat but is it really worth it? We need to look beyond weight loss and consider our total health and vitality. Besides, could you eat like this forever? Neither could most people, according to much of the research to date. Such diets work in the short term, but over 12 months they perform no better than any other diet.

While it may be better than the previous two diets, you can see that the fitness junkie's diet shown in Figure 8.3 is still lacking in some areas. Highly processed protein drinks and low-fat lollies are common treats while fruits, because they provide carbohydrates, are frowned upon

No surprises here. The fast-food junkie's diet, shown in Figure 8.4 is bottom of the league where almost every player is a liability! We need say no more. Figure 8.5 shows what to strive for. This is your 'winning team'. If, most of the time, you select from the star and 5-star performing foods, you will look, feel and perform at your very best.

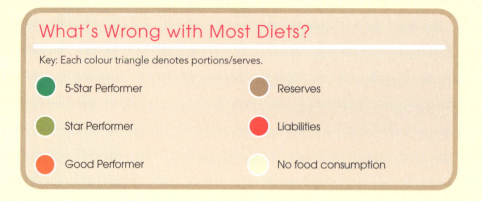

What's Wrong with Most Diets?

Key: Each colour triangle denotes portions/serves.

- 5-Star Performer
- Star Performer
- Good Performer
- Reserves
- Liabilities
- No food consumption

THE LOW-FAT DIET

★ Missing essential good fats
★ Too many sugary low-fat treats
★ Too many high-GI carbohydrates

THE HIGH PROTEIN DIET

★ Insufficient vegetable and no fruit
★ Not enough fibre
★ Too much saturated fat

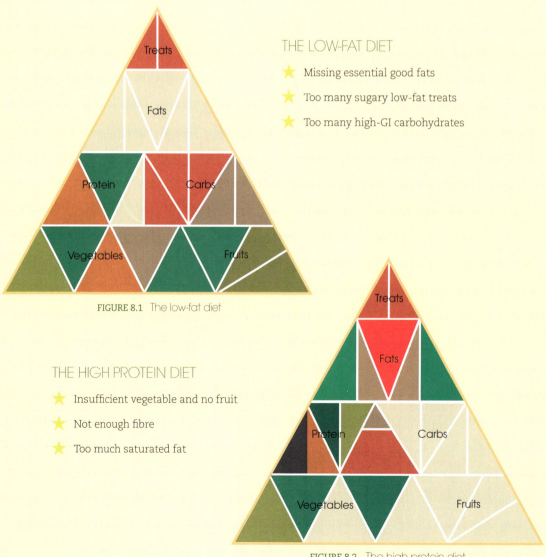

FIGURE 8.1 The low-fat diet

FIGURE 8.2 The high-protein diet

THE FITNESS JUNKIE

★ Insufficient carbohydrate to support exercise

★ Too many sugary low-fat treats

★ Relies on processed protein supplements

FIGURE 8.3 The fitness junkie

THE FAST-FOOD JUNKIE

★ Poor quality carbohydrate, protein and fat

★ Insufficient vegetable and fruit

★ Too many treats

FIGURE 8.4 The fast-food junkie

THE WINNING TEAM

★ Best quality carbohydrate protein and fat

★ Rich in micronutrients and phytochemicals

★ Enjoys quality treats in moderation

FIGURE 8.5 The winning team

The new you!

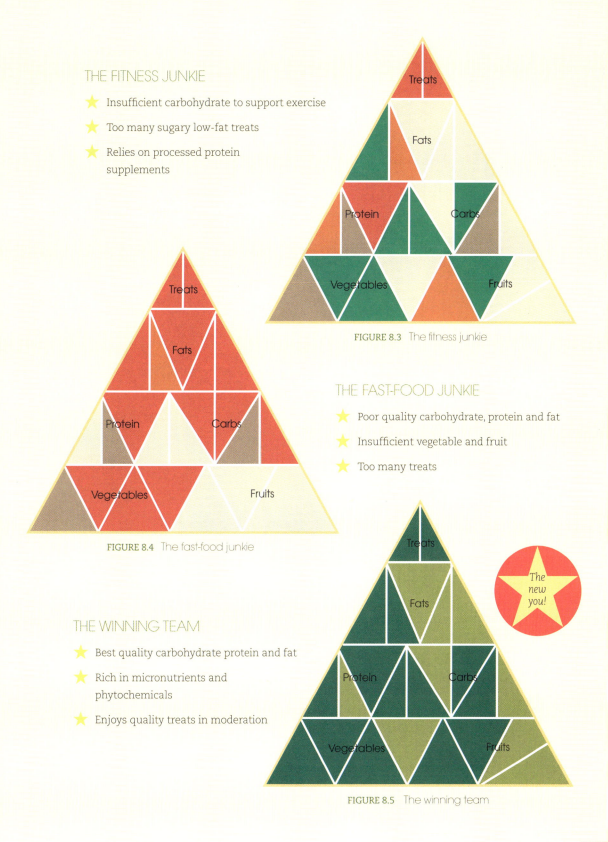

What's Wrong with Most Diets?

Chapter 9

Cooking and Recipes

If you regard cooking as a chore it always will be. If you see it as a creative expression you may see yourself as an artist. It's a better option than feeling like a slave to the kitchen and servant to those you cook for. Best of all, what you cook will taste much better.

I didn't train as a chef or learn how to cook at school. I write this to anyone who has reached this section of the book and is now saying it's too hard to cook and you simply don't have the time to do it. I learned to cook because I like eating and I like eating good food. Being vain and with a tendency to gain fat, I started with the desire to eat the types of food that helped maintain my body size. And I felt better for it.

Now in my 40s, I want to stay fit and active and as young looking as possible. Were I in my 50s I might be saying I wanted to avoid chronic disease, and in my 60s I'll probably be saying I want to reach a grand old age. Whatever your motivation is, the facts are you'll feel better at any age if you make a choice to get into the kitchen and learn how to prepare easy, healthy meals using fresh natural ingredients.

Suspend disbelief about your ability in the kitchen and recognise that anyone can learn anything with a little invested time and practice. With that on board, it's handy to know that most modern recipes, including the majority in this recipe section, can be made in around 30 minutes—less time than it would take for a home delivery meal to arrive!

The tricks of a healthy eater

If you've been a 'reserve or liability' eater most of your days you have a bit of work to do but, like any new learning that requires effort and usually involves making a number of mistakes, what starts off feeling difficult and uncomfortable will in time become surprisingly simple.

Here are the tricks of the healthy eater.

OUT WITH THE OLD

With your food hierarchies as a guide, go through your refrigerator and freezer and throw out all the 'reserve and liability' foods. And, if you order take away most nights of the week, throw the menus out as well.

THE BASIC TOOLS TO MAKE COOKING EASIER

You don't have to buy an entire kitchen collection but there are some basics you do need to get food on the table quickly and efficiently, and they needn't cost you a fortune.

Check the list of kitchen items below and stock up with the things you don't have:

Item	Why you need it	✓
2 baking trays	To roast veggies etc.	
1 baking sheet	To finish off meat and fish.	
Chargrill pan	To sear/grill meat, fish and veggies.	
2 chopping boards	One for veggies and fruit the other for meat and fish.	
Sieve	For draining grains and veggies.	
Food processor	The quickest way to make sauces and pastry, and blend soups.	
Heavy-based oven-proof frying pan with lid	For stove top and oven cooking, to sauté and make hearty casseroles.	
Garlic press	A great time saver.	
Jar with lid	Any jar will do to make and mix salad dressings in.	
Multi-size grater	Large holes for cheese, veggies, smaller holes for ginger, Parmesan, nutmeg.	
Knives	No compromise here—a couple of good quality knives make an enormous difference in the kitchen. Ideally you want a large heavy multi-purpose blade, a smaller knife to use on small items, and a small serrated blade for trimming around veggies and fruit peel.	
Ladle	Useful for soups and soupy casseroles.	
Measuring spoons and cups	There's less need to measure most 5-star performers but, in some recipes, if you don't they'll either not taste so great or won't work. Besides, a careless extra slurp of olive oil amounts to an additional 673 unnecessary kilojoules; less than useful when you want to lose weight.	
Mixing bowls	A set of stainless steel bowls are everyday musts; used to mix grains for breakfast cereal, toss salad leaves, beat eggs etc.	
Salad spinner	This will sway those who skip the salad on the side because they can't be bothered washing and drying the greens. With salad greens washed and dried in seconds and a dressing whipped up in a couple of minutes, a side salad will become part of everyday eating.	
Scissors	Handy to open plastic sealed packaging.	
Large slotted spoon	To remove poached eggs, also very handy when serving thick chunky veggie soup.	
Small pancake or omelette pan	Handy for dry roasting nuts and seeds, and (obviously) making omelettes and pancakes!	
Spatula	Essential.	
Stainless steel saucepans	Buy quality pans—a large stockpot for pasta and soups, a medium pan and a small pan are a good basic starting kit.	
Steamer	Buy a stainless steel steamer to fit on one of your pans. A bamboo steamer is another cheaper alternative.	
Tongs	Forget the long tongs which give you no control whatsoever; a small pair to turn meat and fish and serve with is essential.	
Vegetable peeler	For the obvious and to make cheese shavings.	
Wok	If your stove is electric, buy an electric wok. For gas users, a large cast-iron wok makes an easy and delicious stir-fry in minutes.	
Wooden spoons	A couple are useful.	

Shopping

There are a number of online websites you can use these days to make shopping easier and faster, but most people still prefer to get out to the shops and select their own fresh produce. It entirely depends on what you can make time for. Ideally, you'll be able to make time for a big shop (usually on the weekend) and a mini shop later in the week to pick up a few extra perishables for the remainder of the week. Fresh fish is best eaten on the day it's bought or at the latest the day after. Meat, provided it's well wrapped, will be fine refrigerated for up to 4 days. If you buy it vacuum packed it lasts even longer. Leafy vegetables, stored in plastic bags in the refrigerator will be good for up to 4 days. Root vegetables and harder vegetables such as sweet potato, onion, carrot and garlic will store in the pantry for a couple of weeks. Here are some more tips:

- ★ Depending on the number of people you're catering for, you should be able to stock up your healthy pantry and fridge with one big shop and one mini shop later in the week.
- ★ On the big shop you'll buy the labour-saving foods and the perishables.
- ★ Labour-saving foods are things like canned tomatoes, canned legumes, canned fish, natural preservative stocks, pasta sauces, condiments such as tamari, tahini, sodium-reduced soy sauce, preserved lemons, oils, vinegar, tea, bottled water, nuts and seeds, mixed grains, dried fruit, herbs and spices, frozen berries and frozen veggies.
- ★ The perishables include fresh meat, fish, low-fat dairy and as much fruit and vegetables to get you by until the next mini shop.
- ★ The mini shop is to top up on the perishable foods to see you through to the end of the week. Depending on the services near you, it may be more enjoyable to do the mini shop at the local shops with a green grocer, butcher and (hopefully) a fish shop and save the large shop for the major shopping centre.

WHEN TO SHOP

If you work Monday to Friday, it may seem like a drag allocating a couple of hours to grocery shopping on one of your valuable days off but, if you do it when you have time to spare, you're more likely to plan properly and less likely to forget anything. You'll also have time to unpack and store your produce properly when you get home. If you get off to an early start, you'll hit the shops before the crowds and have the rest of the day to eat well and have fun.

Don't panic—you won't have to go grocery shopping every Saturday or Sunday for the rest of your days. In time the process will become easier, and you'll master it sufficiently to whip around the shops in half the time.

Farmers markets, fish markets and food provedores make buying fresh produce a great day out so it's well worth investigating what's going on in your area.

Breakfasts

Some people say breakfast is their favourite meal of the day. Observing them, they're generally slim, full of energy, glowing with health, and positive. Others say they don't feel like eating first thing in the morning. Observing them, they're often none of the things described above.

Research backs up these observations, particularly in relation to weight control—breakfast eaters are indeed slimmer. Whether you have to eat less or earlier at night, or get up earlier to exercise so you build an appetite, it's worth doing. Breakfast is the meal that breaks the fast from the long night's sleep. It boosts the metabolism, gives you the energy to get through the morning's activities and helps you maintain focus and attention.

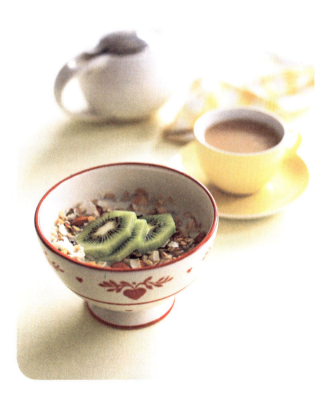

Triple Grain Muesli *Serves 20*

It's unlikely you'll ever find prunes in commercial muesli because they all tend to clump together if they're chopped in an electric processor. You'll have to chop them by hand and add them to the grain a few at a time. It's also worth making your own LSA (ground linseeds, sunflower seeds and almonds) rather than buying it from a health food store. It's fresher and the texture is less like sand. Grind it just long enough to break up the seeds but keep the almonds crunchy. It might seem like a chore to make your own muesli, but it really is worth the effort. At the end of the day, you've made a delicious premium muesli where every single ingredient rates as a 5-star performer.

Ingredients

- 1 cup raw almonds
- 1 cup sunflower seeds
- 1 cup linseeds (flaxseeds)
- 2 cups rolled oats
- 2 cups rolled barley flakes
- 2 cups rolled rye flakes
- ½ cup dried apricots, roughly chopped
- 1 cup pitted prunes, roughly chopped

Method

1. Grind the almonds, sunflower seeds and linseeds in a food processor.
2. Combine with the rolled grains. Add the dried fruit slowly and stir through as you go to prevent the fruit clumping together.
3. Store in the refrigerator in an airtight container.
4. Serve with fresh fruit, low fat natural yoghurt and linseed (flaxseed) oil.

A Slight Break from Tradition—Porridge *Serves 4*

Traditional Scottish porridge is made with coarse oats, water and salt, although no-one I know likes it like that (except Joanna's Mum!). Nowadays porridge is made using a variety of oats including rolled oats, quick oats and instant oats. The less processed oats are, the lower the GI of the porridge is. Therefore, while it may take longer to cook, porridge made from coarse oats is the healthiest choice. By breaking from tradition with added ginger, fruit and nuts, we create a far more interesting and delicious meal with numerous health attributes in addition to those from oats alone. This dish can be made in the slow cooker and cooked overnight.

Ingredients

1 cup coarse oats
1½ litres water
1 tablespoon grated fresh ginger
1 green apple cut into rough chunks
1 teaspoon sea salt
1 cup low-fat milk
2 tablespoons walnuts
1 tablespoon pepitas (pumpkin seeds)
6 dried apricots finely chopped

Method

1. Soak the oats in water overnight.
2. Drain thoroughly and place the oats in a pan with the water, ginger, apple and sea salt.
3. Bring to the boil nd then reduce the heat to simmer for 50 minutes stirring occasionally until most of the water has absorbed and the grain is soft.
4. Add the low-fat milk, nuts, seeds and apricots and stir through.

Tip: Delicious served with fresh fruit and a tablespoon of honey and soy or low-fat milk or yoghurt.

Chachouka *Serves 4*

This Middle Eastern dish is a little left of centre from traditional breakfast fodder, but I love finding opportunities to boost veggie intake and kick-start the metabolism with some spices.

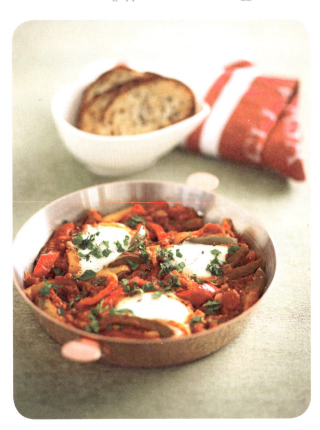

Ingredients

2 tablespoons camellia tea oil

1 clove garlic, crushed

1 small red chilli, deseeded and finely chopped

1 brown onion, chopped

½ teaspoon ground cumin

1 teaspoon sweet paprika

1 400 g can organic tomatoes, chopped

⅓ cup water

2 red capsicums, cut into strips

1 yellow capsicum, cut into strips

1 green capsicum, cut into strips

4 free range eggs

Method

1. Heat the oil in a pan over medium heat and add the garlic, chilli, onion, cumin and paprika.
2. Sauté for 2 minutes.
3. Add the chopped tomatoes, water and capsicums and cook until the capsicums are soft.
4. Form 4 indents in the mix and crack an egg into each one.
5. Cook with the lid on the pan until the egg is cooked through (approximately 10 minutes).
6. Serve on a piece of toasted wholegrain/spelt bread.

Notes: Some people experience digestive irritation with capsicum. This may be minimised by removing the skin or avoiding the unripe varieties (yellow and green).

A recent survey found that 68 per cent of capsicums were found to contain pesticides so it may be worth paying more for organic when you can (Fenoll et al, 2007).

Strawberry Breakfast Trifle *Serves 4*

Here's an excellent start to the day—if you don't have a sweet tooth you can omit the maple syrup, particularly if the strawberries are sweet. Children may find it more approachable with the syrup added and, if it helps them eat oats and seeds, it's well worth adding.

Ingredients

2 cups rolled oats
2 tablespoons almonds
2 tablespoons sunflower seeds
2 tablespoons pepitas (pumpkin seeds)
2 tablespoons maple syrup
1 large punnet strawberries, washed, hulled and cut into quarters
220 g low-fat natural yoghurt

Method

1. Preheat oven to 180°C.
2. Coat the oats, nuts and seeds with maple syrup and lay out on a flat baking sheet lined with baking paper.
3. Place in the middle of the oven and dry-roast for approximately 8 minutes, turning them regularly with a spoon to prevent them from burning.
4. Remove from the oven and set aside.
5. In a glass dish, arrange a layer of strawberries on the bottom, then a layer of the oat and seed mixture, and top with natural yoghurt, repeat the process finishing with a few strawberries to garnish.

Breakfast Quinoa *Serves 4–6*

Many commercial gluten-free breakfast cereals have a high GI. This breakfast quinoa is suitable for people who can't eat wheat and/or gluten and it also has a low GI to sustain energy throughout the morning. Apple juice concentrate is a natural sweetener available from health food stores.

Ingredients

2 cups quinoa
2½ cups cold water
1 cinnamon stick
½ cup apple juice concentrate
½ cup mixed chopped nuts (almonds, Brazil nuts, walnuts)
¼ cup dried apricots, chopped
fresh fruit or stewed fruit compote, to serve
low-fat natural yoghurt, to serve

Method

1. Thoroughly rinse and drain the quinoa.
2. Add to a pan with the water, cinnamon stick and apple concentrate and bring to the boil. Reduce to simmer and cover.
3. Cook for 15 minutes until the quinoa is tender and the liquid has absorbed into the grain.
4. While the quinoa is cooking, dry-roast the nuts in a frying pan until they're golden and fragrant.
5. Stir the nuts and chopped apricots through the quinoa and serve with fresh or stewed fruit and yoghurt.
6. This will store for up to 3 days in the refrigerator.

Buckwheat Pancakes with Blueberry Sauce and Bush Honey Yoghurt *Serves 6*

Here's a nice breakfast for the whole family to enjoy. Even though berries are not in season during winter, you can always use frozen—nutritionally they're just as good and much cheaper.

Ingredients

2 punnets blueberries
4 tablespoons bush honey
1 tablespoon lemon juice
¾ cup buckwheat flour
¼ cup wholemeal flour, sifted
sea salt
2 free range eggs

1½ cups buttermilk
½ cup water
1½ cups low-fat plain yoghurt
olive or grapeseed oil
1 punnet strawberries, to serve
1 punnet raspberries, to serve

Method

1. In a small pan, slowly bring a punnet of blueberries to the boil with 1 tablespoon water, 2 tablespoons honey and the lemon juice. Cover and reduce the heat to a slow simmer for 3 minutes until the berries have stewed.
2. Mix in a blender until quite smooth.
3. Sift the flours and a pinch of sea salt into a bowl. Make a well in the centre and add the eggs. Beat the eggs into the flour.
4. Gradually add the buttermilk and water and beat until bubbles form on the surface of the pancake batter. Cover and refrigerate until ready to use.
5. Add the remaining honey to the yoghurt, beat together and refrigerate.
6. Using kitchen paper and olive or grapeseed oil, lightly oil a small pancake pan.
7. Beat the pancake mixture once again before transferring into a jug for easy pouring.
8. Pour enough batter into the pan to cover the bottom and make a pancake approximately 4 mm thick.
9. Cook for approximately 3–4 minutes or until bubbles form on the surface of the pancake.
10. Flip the pancake and cook for a further minute.
11. Repeat the process until the batter mix is finished.
12. Serve with berries, topped with yoghurt and honey sauce.

Entrées and Light Meals

Even if you're not that hungry at mealtimes, you should still make the effort to make a light meal incorporating a few 5-star performing ingredients. It's another opportunity to feed your body the nutrients it needs to power through the day. Compared to eating one or two large meals, eating more frequent smaller meals helps you to manage your weight better and gives your body a chance to absorb all those wonderful nutrients across the course of the day rather than being bombarded with an enormous load all at once. The latter is likely to leave you lethargic, bloated and, if late at night, unable to sleep well.

5-star performing foods—raw nuts, olive oil

Spicy Roast Nuts Serves 4–6

These nuts make a nice snack to serve with pre-dinner drinks. They're much healthier than commercial varieties and, when served warm, much more delicious.

Ingredients

1 cup mixed raw nuts (include cashews, almonds, walnuts and Brazil nuts)
½ tablespoon olive oil
½ teaspoon fine sea salt
pinch chilli flakes

Method

1 Preheat the oven to 200°C.

2 Line a baking tray with baking paper.

3 Lay the nuts on the sheet and sprinkle the olive oil over them, shaking them gently on the tray to ensure each nut is lightly coated with oil.

4 Sprinkle sea salt and chilli flakes over them and stir through.

5 Place the tray in the oven and roast for 4–5 minutes. Stir through to allow them to roast evenly and roast for a further 4 minutes.

Note: Nuts can turn rancid or mouldy if they've been stored too long or left unsealed in a warm place. To avoid rancidity, and the risk of free radical damage from eating rancid nuts, buy raw nuts and store them in a sealed jar in the refrigerator.

Avocado Gazpacho *Serves 6*

Packed with top-performing ingredients, this cold soup can also be used as a dressing over salad greens and fresh prawns. Store in the refrigerator for up to 5 days in an airtight container.

Ingredients

3 small ripe avocados
1 Lebanese cucumber, roughly chopped
1 green capsicum, deseeded
1 green chilli, deseeded
1 Spanish (red) onion, peeled
2 cloves garlic, peeled
2 cups cold, filtered water
1 teaspoon sea salt
1 bunch coriander
juice of 1 lime
cracked black pepper

To serve

½ cup low-fat plain yoghurt
pinch smoked paprika
limes, quartered

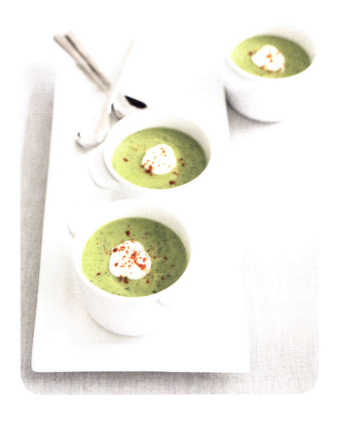

Method

1. Skin, halve and stone avocados.
2. Using a juicer, juice the cucumber, capsicum, chilli, onion and garlic.
3. Combine the vegetable juice, avocados, water, salt, coriander, lime juice and black pepper in a blender and process thoroughly.
4. Serve chilled, with a dollop of low-fat plain yoghurt, a sprinkle of smoked paprika, lime quarters and cracked pepper.

Tip: If you don't use a whole avocado straight away, replace the seed, sprinkle the exposed flesh with lemon juice and wrap it tightly in foil before refrigerating. Eat within 1 to 2 days of cutting.

Shiitake and Buckwheat Soup *Serves 6*

This rich-tasting soup is an excellent winter warmer. In Eastern medicine, shiitake mushrooms are reputed to have immune-boosting qualities—another bonus during the season in which we're most prone to bacterial and viral attack.

Ingredients

8 shiitake mushrooms
2 cups hot water
6 cups water, extra
¼ cup buckwheat
2 whole shallots
1 × 3 cm piece ginger, peeled
2 star anise
3 tablespoons mirin
3 tablespoons tamari
1 carrot, julienned
4 shallots, finely chopped, extra
½ bunch coriander, chopped

Method

1. Place shiitake mushrooms in a bowl and cover with 2 cups hot water. Allow to stand for 20 minutes.
2. Add the soaking water to a saucepan with 6 cups water, buckwheat, whole shallots, ginger, star anise, mirin and tamari.
3. Bring to the boil slowly and simmer for 20 minutes.
4. Add the carrots and sliced shiitake (stems removed) and cook for a further 15 minutes.
5. Remove ginger, shallots and star anise.
6. Place into serving bowls and add 1 teaspoon each chopped coriander and chopped shallots.

Vegetarian San Choy Bau Serves 4–6

I challenge people who say they don't like tofu. It's a bit like art and music—you're bound to like some version of it. Most people object to the texture and the fact that it doesn't taste of anything. However, this can work to your advantage as tofu will take on the flavours you wish it to in the dish. This recipe does just that and disguises the texture so much some people could even be fooled into thinking they were eating meat.

Ingredients

350 g firm tofu
2 tablespoons pine nuts
1 tablespoon olive oil
300 g cup mushrooms, finely chopped
1 red chilli, finely chopped
3 coriander roots, scrubbed and crushed
2 tablespoons salt-reduced soy sauce
4 shallots, thinly sliced
juice of ½ lemon
¼ bunch coriander leaves
½ savoy cabbage

Method

1. Cut the tofu into cubes and place in a pan filled with water.
2. Bring the water to the boil, reduce the heat slightly and cook until the tofu rises to the surface of the water.
3. Drain the water, blot the tofu dry and place in a food processor.
4. Mince the tofu into small pieces.
5. In a small pan, dry-roast the pine nuts until golden taking care not to burn them. Remove from the heat and set aside.
6. Heat wok over a high heat until hot before adding the oil, mushrooms, chilli and crushed coriander root. Stir-fry for 4 minutes.
7. Add the minced tofu and stir-fry for a further 2 minutes. Add the soy sauce and most of the shallots (reserving some for garnishing).
8. Stir through the lemon juice, pine nuts and coriander leaves.
9. Carefully separate the cabbage leaves trying to keep them whole. Steam the leaves in a bamboo steamer for 5 minutes.
10. Fill each cabbage leaf with the tofu mixture. Top with chopped shallots and, if desired, extra soy sauce for seasoning.

5-star performing foods—sardines, lemon, olive oil, garlic, wholegrain bread, avocado, capsicum

Sardine, Avocado and Capsicum Grill *Serves 4*

Here's an easy and substantial meal that tastes great and is packed with nutritional goodies.

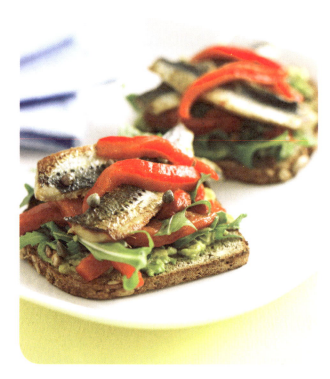

Ingredients

12 sardine fillets

olive oil

juice of ½ lemon

4 slices wholegrain bread, toasted

1 avocado

2 tablespoons capers

black pepper

1 cup rocket leaves

1 roast capsicum, sliced

Method

1. Brush the sardines with olive oil and a sprinkle of lemon juice.
2. Heat a grill pan and cook sardines for 3–4 minutes on one side only.
3. Spread each slice of toast with avocado and sprinkle the capers over the top. Season with black pepper and a little more lemon juice.
4. Lay the rocket over the avocado.
5. Top with sardines and sliced capsicum and serve.

Oysters with Diced Vegetables and Herb Vinaigrette *Serves 4*

Natural oysters with a squeeze of lemon juice and black pepper are delicious but, to boost the nutritional value a little more, try chopping a few veggies and herbs over them too.

Ingredients

1 small carrot
1 stick celery
¼ red capsicum
¼ green capsicum
1 tablespoon chopped basil
1 tablespoon chopped chervil
3 tablespoons extra virgin cold pressed olive oil
1 tablespoon lemon juice
24 oysters
cracked black pepper

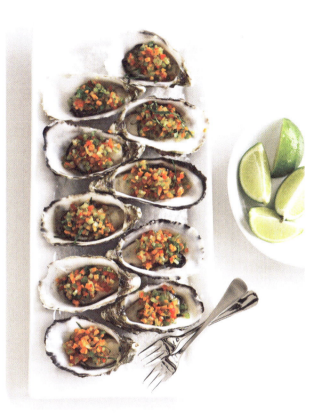

Method

1. Finely dice the carrot, celery and capsicums. Place in a bowl with the chopped herbs.
2. Stir through the olive oil and lemon juice.
3. Serve a spoonful of the vegetable mixture on each oyster.
4. Season with cracked black pepper.

Opening oysters

If you're lucky enough to come across an oyster farm selling oysters direct to the public, it's worth knowing how to open them and avoid injury.

Fold a cloth several times and lay it in the palm of your left hand (right if you're left handed). Hold the oyster firmly in the cloth flat side facing up. Take a short bladed oyster knife to prise between the hinged side separating the closing muscle. Move the knife flat across the oyster and use it as a lever to separate the two halves.

Poached Eggs with Asparagus and Shaved Goat's Cheese *Serves 2*

This is a perfect dish to serve in the evening if you've had a large lunch—it's extremely quick to prepare and make, and is satisfying yet not too heavy.

Ingredients

1 tablespoon white vinegar
4 free range eggs
1 bunch fresh asparagus, trimmed and washed
30 gm semi-hard goat's cheese
black pepper

Method

1. Bring a deep frying pan filled with water to the boil.
2. Add 1 tablespoon vinegar to the water and reduce to simmer.
3. Crack the eggs, one at a time, into a small teacup and gently lower the egg into the water. Simmer for 4–5 minutes depending on how you like your eggs.
4. While the eggs are cooking, steam the asparagus for 3–4 minutes.
5. Remove from the heat. Lay the asparagus on a dinner plate.
6. Using a slotted spoon, ease each egg from the water and let the water drain away.
7. Arrange the eggs on top of the asparagus then, using a potato peeler, shave the goat's cheese over the top.
8. Season with cracked black pepper and serve

> **Tip**: *Always use very fresh eggs when poaching.*

Cucumber, Eggplant, Avocado and Bulgur Timbale *Serves 4*

This impressive looking dish is a fabulous entrée at any dinner party. It's delicious served on its own with the dressing recipe as shown or with the Avocado Gazpacho (recipe page 153). If you don't have a metal ring, don't worry—on its own as a 'free' salad it's still great.

Ingredients

½ cup coarse bulgur

1 cup boiling water

1 small eggplant, finely diced

juice of 1 lemon

2 Lebanese cucumbers

½ cup chopped parsley

4 vine-ripened tomatoes, peeled, deseeded and chopped

1 avocado, diced

30 ml olive oil

10 ml white balsamic vinegar

1 teaspoon Dijon mustard

1 large clove garlic

Method

1. Rinse the bulgur thoroughly then leave it to soak in a bowl with 1 cup boiling water.
2. Finely dice the eggplant and sprinkle the lemon juice over it. Cover and set aside.
3. Drain any excess moisture from the bulgur and combine it with the cucumber, parsley and tomato.
4. Lay a large metal ring on a plate and fill it with one-quarter of the bulgur and vegetable mix. Top with chopped avocado.
5. Remove the ring and repeat until you have completed 4.
6. Combine the olive oil, vinegar, mustard and garlic and drizzle a spoonful over each timbale.

Mediterranean Mussels *Serves 4*

They're inexpensive to buy, loaded with iron and make a delicious meal, particularly served with a grainy sourdough and side salad.

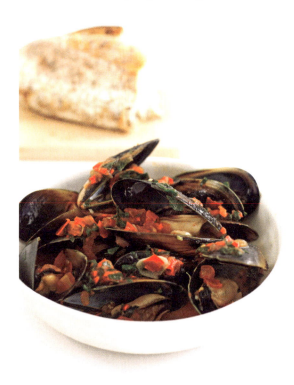

Ingredients

1 tablespoon olive oil
4 cloves garlic, finely sliced
2 large red chillies, finely chopped
4 vine-ripened tomatoes, chopped
1 cup fish stock
2 kg mussels, scrubbed and debearded
1 bunch parsley, chopped
cracked black pepper

Method

1 In a large pan with a lid, place the olive oil, garlic and chilli and sauté for 2 minutes.

2 Add the tomatoes and fish stock and bring the liquid slowly to the boil.

3 Add the mussels and parsley and cover and cook for approximately 5 minutes until the mussels have opened. (Discard any mussels that don't open.)

4 Season with black pepper and serve.

Mussels

Australian Blue mussels are a sustainable seafood and a better choice than imported New Zealand Green mussels. They should always be bought fresh and cooked on the day they are bought. Select tightly closed shells or, if slightly open, those that snap shut when tapped. Those that are open are dead and should be discarded. Store them in a damp cloth in the refrigerator, as plastic will suffocate the live mussel. Scrub the shells clean using a bristle brush or abrasive cloth. Mussels attach themselves to rocks with their beards and these must be removed before cooking. This is easily achieved by grabbing the beard that is hanging out of the shell with fingers or fine-pointed pliers and pulling it out in the direction of the hinged end of the shell.

Lentil and Freekeh Patties with Coleslaw *Serves 4*

The vegetarians and vegans among you will have to fight your meat-eating friends for a share of these lentil patties. They're a great source of protein and fibre, boosted by combining the grain freekeh with the lentils, and they have a low GI.

Patties

½ cup whole freekeh

1 cup brown lentils

3 cups water

1 tablespoon olive oil

1 small brown onion, peeled and finely chopped

2 cloves garlic

2 teaspoons cumin

2 teaspoons ground coriander powder

2 pieces preserved lemon or lime, pulp removed and skin finely chopped

⅓ cup chopped coriander

sea salt and ground black pepper to season

Coleslaw

1 carrot, grated

2 shallots, sliced

2 cups finely sliced green cabbage

1 cup finely sliced red cabbage

1 cup grated red radish

1 cup sheep's yoghurt

2 tablespoons lime juice

1 teaspoon maple syrup

1 avocado

cut limes, to serve

Method

1. Cook the freekeh according to the instructions on the packet.
2. While the grain is cooking, in a separate pan, add the lentils, 3 cups water, and bring to the boil. Reduce the heat and simmer for approximately 30 minutes until the lentils are tender.
3. Drain the freekeh and lentils of any excess water.
4. Place in a food processor and process until they are well combined but retain texture.
5. Heat the olive oil in a small pan.
6. Add the onions and garlic and sauté for a couple of minutes until tender.
7. Add the spices and cook for a further 2 minutes.
8. Transfer the onion mix to a bowl with the lentil and freekeh mixture.
9. Combine thoroughly with preserved lemon, fresh coriander and seasoning.
10. Mould the mixture into flat patties (approx 8 cm × 2.5 cm).
11. Heat a non-stick pan with one tablespoon of olive oil and pan-fry the patties for 3–4 minutes each side.
12. To make the coleslaw, combine the vegetables in a bowl.
13. Mix the yoghurt, lime juice and maple syrup in a separate bowl to make a dressing and combine thoroughly through the coleslaw.
14. Serve over the patties with accompanying slices of fresh avocado and lime juice.

Salads

We've come a long way from shredded iceberg lettuce, tomato quarters and a few slices of thick cucumber. Be adventurous with the salad leaves you use; all have different nutrients, tastes and textures to offer us. Mesclun, the name given to a mix of salad leaves, is usually available in most greengrocers and is a good way of including a range of leaves without buying each individually. Rocket, baby spinach, endive, mignonette, tatsoi and watercress are just a few of the many leaves available.

A salad can be a meal in itself or an accessory to a main meal. The secret to green salad is choosing a variety of fresh green leaves and serving them in a beautiful shallow bowl. It doesn't have to resemble a supreme pizza with 101 ingredients added. Less is often best.

5-star performing foods—dark salad greens, extra virgin camellia tea oil, garlic

Asian Salad *Serves 4*

Ingredients

4 cups mixed greens
⅓ cup extra virgin camellia tea oil
1 tablespoon mirin
1 tablespoon brown rice vinegar
½ tablespoon tamari
1 clove garlic, peeled

Tip: *Invest in a salad spinner if you haven't already. It saves time and ensures veggies and salad greens are thoroughly washed and dried.*

Method

1. Wash and dry the salad greens and place in a mixing bowl.
2. Combine the oil, mirin, brown rice vinegar and tamari in a small jar.
3. Gently press the flat edge of a knife on the garlic clove to slightly bruise it before dropping it into the jar.
4. Seal and shake the jar to combine the ingredients and set aside for about 30 minutes.
5. Discard the garlic.
6. Shake the jar again and toss the dressing over the leaves.

Note: 1 cup salad greens is the equivalent to 1 serve. If you're at the greengrocer buying greens from the salad basket, estimate two tong scoops per person.

Quinoa Tabbouleh *Serves 6*

Bulgur is typically used to make tabbouleh and is another of our star performer grains. For those who suffer a wheat/gluten intolerance or allergy, this version using quinoa is a terrific alternative.

Ingredients

2 cups quinoa, cooked and cooled (see instruction below)
2 cups chopped parsley
¼ bunch mint, chopped roughly
¼ bunch rocket, chopped roughly
3 vine-ripened tomatoes, deseeded and chopped
juice of 1 lemon
¼ cup extra virgin olive oil
3 cloves garlic, crushed
1 teaspoon sumac
cracked black pepper

Method

1. Cook the quinoa (1 cup quinoa to 2 cups water; bring to the boil; reduce the heat and cover; simmer for 10–15 minutes.)
2. Set cooked quinoa aside on a flat dish, spreading it out to allow it to cool evenly.
3. When quinoa is cool, combine all ingredients and serve.

Fatoush *Serves 4*

Fatoush is a Middle Eastern dish, traditionally made with pita bread. The bread has been substituted here with sesame seeds. The sesame loads the dish up with more star fats and, in my opinion, makes it much tastier.

Serve as a companion to lamb or chicken with a spoonful of hummus.

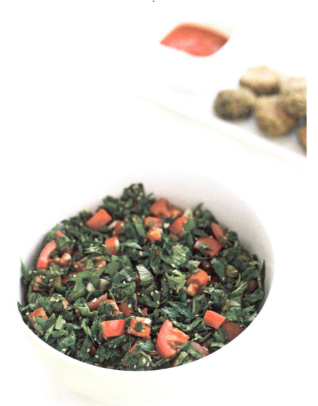

Ingredients

1 tablespoon sesame seeds
1 large bunch flat leaf parsley, roughly chopped
½ bunch mint, roughly chopped
1 bunch baby rocket, roughly chopped
6 shallots, finely sliced
3 vine-ripened tomatoes, roughly chopped
2 Lebanese cucumbers, finely chopped
3 tablespoons capers, drained and rinsed
juice of 1 lemon
2 cloves garlic, crushed
3 tablespoons extra virgin olive oil
1 tablespoon sumac

Method

1. Dry-roast the sesame seeds in a pan over medium heat until they turn slightly golden. Set aside to cool.
2. Place the prepared greens in a bowl with the shallots, tomato and cucumber.
3. Chop the capers finely and add them to the bowl.
4. Combine the lemon juice, garlic, olive oil and sumac in a small bowl, pour it over the salad and toss until the ingredients are well combined.

Note: Sumac is a spice that comes from the ripe berries of a Middle Eastern tree. The berries are harvested, partly dried, then ground to remove the purple–red, tangy flesh from the inner seed. The flavour is tangy, lemon-like, salty and pleasantly acidic. Available from speciality spice stores.

Avocado Mango and Pine Nut Salad *Serves 4*

This is perfect for a dinner party. It can be made in minutes just before you and your guests sit down to eat. Dry-roast the pine nuts and make the dressing in advance.

Ingredients

4 tablespoons pine nuts
3 tablespoons extra virgin cold pressed olive oil
1 tablespoon white balsamic vinegar
½ teaspoon Dijon mustard
2 avocados, peeled and sliced
2 mangos, peeled and sliced
black pepper, to season

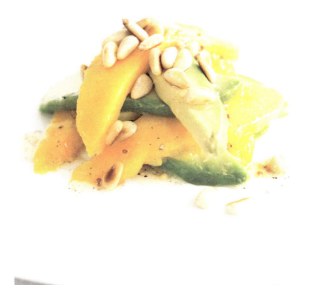

Method

1. In a small dry frying pan, dry-roast the pine nuts over a medium heat until slightly toasted. Set aside to cool.
2. Mix the oil, vinegar and mustard together.
3. Arrange avocado and mango slices on individual plates.
4. Drizzle a tablespoon of dressing over each, season with pepper and top with pine nuts.

Green Salad with Avocado, Almond and Mustard Dressing *Serves 4*

While it's true with so many good fats this salad is higher in kilojoules than many others, it's so good for you that it's better to cut kilojoules in other ways or increase the exercise than go without.

Ingredients

4 cups mixed greens
½ cup chopped flat leaf parsley
¼ cup slivered almonds
3 tablespoons extra virgin olive oil
1 tablespoon white wine vinegar
1 teaspoon wholegrain mustard
cracked black pepper
pinch sea salt
1 large avocado, sliced

Method

1. Wash and dry the salad greens and parsley and place them in a mixing bowl.
2. In a small pan, dry-roast the slivered almonds over a medium heat until they turn golden and fragrant.
3. Combine the oil, vinegar, mustard and seasoning in a small jar.
4. Pour all but 1 teaspoon of the dressing over the leaves.
5. Toss the leaves and arrange them in a serving dish.
6. Arrange the avocado over the leaves, sprinkle the remaining dressing over and top with the almond slivers.

Note: It often happens that a beautiful looking salad is spoilt after the dressing is tossed through it. All the small bits drop to the bottom of the bowl and, if you try to retrieve them, the leaves get knocked about and bruised. The trick to keeping the salad beautiful is to toss the greens with most of the dressing in a large bowl other than the one you're planning to serve the salad in. Once dressed, place them in the serving bowl and top with the other salad items. Then, with a teaspoon, drizzle the remaining dressing over the undressed ingredients.

Grilled Goat's Cheese, Hazelnut and Cranberry Salad *Serves 4*

This dish makes a light lunch or entrée.

Ingredients

4 slices wholegrain sourdough bread
200 g soft goat's cheese
4 teaspoons extra virgin olive oil
large bunch mixed green salad leaves, washed and dried
½ cup roasted hazelnuts
½ cup cranberry sauce
cracked black pepper

Method

1. Toast the bread on one side only under a grill.
2. Remove the bread and lay a couple of pieces of goat's cheese on the untoasted side of each slice.
3. Drizzle each slice with a teaspoon of olive oil and return to the grill for a further 2–3 minutes.
4. Arrange the salad greens on individual plates, top with the hazelnuts.
5. Lay the toast and goat's cheese on the bed of greens, and serve each with a teaspoonful of cranberry sauce and a sprinkling of cracked pepper.

Chargrilled Sesame Octopus and Watercress Salad *Serves 4*

If you don't eat much red meat, it's good to remember that octopus is a great source of iron.

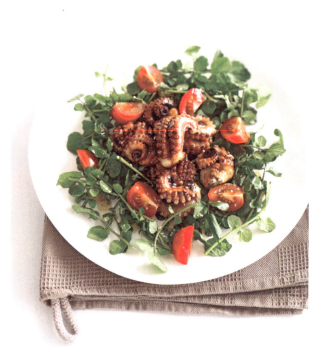

Ingredients

2 tablespoons sesame oil
1 tablespoon lime juice
1 red eye chilli, finely chopped
1 kg baby octopus, washed and trimmed into small pieces
bunch watercress, washed and trimmed
150 g cherry tomatoes, washed

Sesame Dressing

1 tablespoon sesame oil
1 tablespoon olive oil
1 tablespoon lime juice
1 teaspoon tamari
1 teaspoon sesame seeds

Method

1. Combine the sesame oil, lime juice and chilli and pour over the octopus.
2. Set aside to marinate for 1 hour.
3. Drain the octopus from the marinade.
4. Heat a grill pan to hot and chargrill the octopus for 3–5 minutes until cooked through.
5. Combine the dressing ingredients in a small jar.
6. Arrange the watercress and tomato on individual plates with the grilled octopus on top.
7. Drizzle with dressing and serve.

Kangaroo Thai Salad *Serves 4*

Ingredients

500 g kangaroo loin fillet
150 g mixed green salad leaves
1 small fennel bulb, finely sliced
2 Lebanese cucumbers, thinly sliced
1 punnet cherry tomatoes, washed
2 tablespoons finely sliced mint leaves
¼ cup coriander leaves
2 tablespoons chopped roasted organic peanuts, to garnish
6 shallots, sliced, to garnish

Dressing

1 small red chilli, deseeded and chopped
2 cloves garlic, crushed
1 tablespoon finely sliced lemongrass
2 tablespoons lime or lemon juice
1 tablespoon fish sauce
1 tablespoon rice syrup

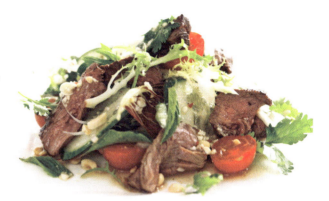

Method

1. Heat an oiled grill pan to very hot.
2. Brown the kangaroo on all sides for approx 6–8 minutes in total.
3. Cover with foil and allow to rest in a warm place for 5 minutes before slicing.
4. Arrange the salad ingredients and herbs on a large platter.
5. Combine the dressing ingredients in a small jar.
6. Once the kangaroo has rested, slice it finely and arrange over the platter.
7. Drizzle the dressing over the meat and salad and sprinkle the chopped peanuts and sliced shallots over the top.

Salmon and Cannellini Bean Salad *Serves 2*

Here's a very easy and healthy lunch to whip up for yourself at home. Make sure you include the bones from the salmon—next to dairy they're the best source of calcium and the crunch factor only adds to the overall dish.

Ingredients

2 cups mixed green salad leaves
1 Lebanese cucumber, sliced
1 carrot, cut into julienne strips
1½ tablespoons extra virgin camellia tea oil
1 tablespoon rice vinegar
½ teaspoon grainy mustard
half a 400 g can cannellini beans
1 x 185 g can red salmon drained with the bones remaining
2 small tomatoes, cut into quarters
cracked black pepper

Method

1. Wash and dry the salad greens. Combine greens with cucumber and carrot.
2. Combine the camellia tea oil, rice vinegar and mustard and toss half of the dressing over the leaves, cucumber and carrots.
3. Drain the cannellini beans and toss the remaining dressing through the beans.
4. Arrange the salad on individual plates.
5. Top with cannellini beans, salmon and tomatoes and season with black pepper.

Note: Left-over cannellini beans are delicious pureéd with olive oil, garlic and a little vinegar. Serve as a low-GI dip or alternative to mashed potatoes or rice.

Chicken and Pomegranate Salad *Serves 4*

The pomegranate gives this chicken salad a fresh sweet, tangy taste.

Ingredients

4 organic chicken breast pieces
1 tablespoon olive oil
100 g raspberries
⅓ cup red wine vinegar
2 tablespoons apple juice concentrate
1 butter lettuce, washed and dried
1 large avocado, peeled and sliced
1 fennel bulb, thinly sliced
2 stalks celery, finely sliced
200 g snow pea sprouts
½ pomegranate, deseeded (cut in half with beads scooped out)

Method

1. Preheat the oven to 180°C.
2. Brush the chicken breasts with olive oil.
3. Chargrill each side of the chicken breasts for 2–3 minutes then place them on a baking tray, covered with foil and cook in the oven for a further 15 minutes or until cooked through.
4. Make the dressing by placing the berries, vinegar and apple juice concentrate in a small saucepan and heating gently for 3 minutes. Blend in a food processor and set aside to cool.
5. Lay the lettuce on a serving plate and arrange the avocado, fennel and celery on top.
6. Slice the chicken and lay it over the salad with the snow pea sprouts and pomegranate seeds over the top.
7. Dress with the raspberry vinaigrette and serve immediately.

Salsas and Sauces

With a few basic salsas and sauces up your sleeve you can create a really interesting dish with some very plain ingredients.

5-star performing foods—tomatoes, olives, onion, chilli, lime

Olive, Coriander, Tomato, Chilli and Lime Salsa Serves 4–6

Take a piece of lean meat, brush it lightly with olive oil, grill it and serve under this salsa and you've created a deliciously tasty meal that's full of flavour and packed with nutrients for very little effort.

Ingredients

6 large vine-ripened tomatoes
½ Spanish (red) onion, peeled and finely chopped
1 small red chilli, deseeded and finely chopped
½ cup pitted kalamata olives, finely chopped
½ bunch coriander (leaves only), roughly chopped
juice of 2 limes
black pepper

Method

1. Using a sharp knife, cut a small cross in the bottom of each tomato. Soak the tomatoes in boiling water until the skin starts to crack and peel. Remove from the boiling water with a slotted spoon. Allow the tomatoes to cool a little so you don't burn yourself, then skin the tomatoes completely. Slice tomatoes in half, remove the seeds and chop the flesh finely.
2. Combine the tomatoes with the onion, chilli, olives and coriander leaves.
3. Add the lime juice and season with black pepper.

Basic Tomato and Basil Sauce   *Makes 4 cups*

The trick to a good pasta sauce is the time taken to cook it—rushed, the sauce will be bitter. There's no need to add sugar when you allow it to simmer slowly for at least 50 minutes. The longer it cooks, the more antioxidants it contains.

Ingredients

3 tablespoons virgin olive oil
1 cup chopped fresh basil
1 small onion, finely chopped
3 cloves garlic, finely chopped
1 small carrot, finely chopped
1 tablespoon finely chopped fresh thyme,
1 tablespoon finely chopped fresh oregano
4 × 400 g cans tomatoes, chopped

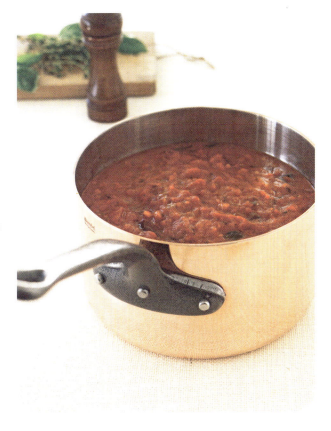

Method

1. Heat the oil in a large saucepan until it's very hot but not smoking.
2. Add the basil and 'deep-fry' for a couple of minutes.
3. Add the onion, garlic, carrot and herbs and sauté until soft.
4. Add the tomatoes and bring to the boil.
5. Reduce the heat and simmer for 50 minutes or until the liquid has thickened and reduced by half.

Cheat's Tip: *If you're buying pasta sauce, check the ingredients and nutritional panel to find one that's made from fresh ingredients and is low in salt and sugar. There are some great ones around and they are excellent to stash away in the pantry in case of an emergency.*

Tip: *Break up whole canned tomatoes with your hands rather than using a metal knife. For some reason, this gives the sauce a richer, less acidic flavour.*

Lime, Corn and Coriander Salsa *Serves 4*

As befitting its Mexican origin, this Mexican corn and lime salsa is equally delicious with spicy beans as it is grilled chicken or fish.

Ingredients

2 cobs sweet corn
juice of 2 limes
1 small Spanish (red) onion, peeled and finely chopped
½ cup coriander leaves, chopped
1 red chilli, deseeded and finely chopped

Method

1. Steam the corn cobs for 3 minutes
2. Once cool, remove the kernels from the cob.
3. Mix the lime juice, Spanish (red) onion, coriander leaves, chilli and corn kernels together in a bowl.
4. Allow the flavours to combine for at least 1 hour before serving.

Walnut Pesto *Makes ½ cup*

This walnut pesto uses fennel in place of Parmesan and cayenne for an extra kick. It's delicious served over grilled fish or chicken and mashed pumpkin, or with slow-roasted tomatoes and pasta.

Ingredients

3 tablespoons raw walnuts, chopped
1 bunch continental parsley
½ cup basil leaves
2 cloves garlic, chopped
1 small piece of fennel, chopped (to make approximately 2 tablespoons)
1 pinch cayenne pepper
juice of ½ lemon
a pinch sea salt
⅓ cup extra virgin olive oil

Method

1. Dry-roast the walnuts in a small flat pan over a medium heat until they have toasted and turned golden brown, approximately 3–4 minutes.
2. In a food processor, place the walnuts, parsley, basil leaves, garlic, fennel, cayenne pepper, lemon juice and sea salt.
3. Process the ingredients, adding the olive oil slowly while the motor is running until the pesto is well combined but not completely smooth. The pesto should still have a granular texture.
4. Store in the refrigerator in an airtight jar ready for use.

Notes: Half a teaspoon of a herb or spice can transform a dish from bland to inspiring. An investment in a few excellent quality herbs and spices is well worth it. To ensure quality and freshness, find a shop with high turnover of produce or, better still, a specialty spice store. To retain freshness, spices should always be stored in airtight containers away from sunlight.

Cayenne

Natural health practitioners believe cayenne is one of the most useful and valuable herbs strengthening the digestive, cardiovascular and circulatory systems.

Side Dishes

The title 'side dish' is not intended to give the impression that these dishes are less important than any of the others. Here you will find a collection of delicious and extremely healthy accessories to dress up the simplest meal. Many may take centre stage in front of the grilled meat or fish they may be served with.

5-star performing foods—broccolini, bok choy, shallots, ginger, garlic, olive oil

Stir-fried Asian Greens Serves 4

Try not to let a single day go by without eating a serve of green leafy vegetables. Here's a very fast and easy way to serve Asian greens. And there's no need to follow the ingredients to the letter here—any variety of greens will work, but try to vary the look and texture to make the dish interesting.

Ingredients

2 tablespoons white sesame seeds
1 bunch broccolini
2 cups snow peas
1 bunch bok choy
½ bunch shallots
½ tablespoon sesame oil
1 tablespoon tamari
2 teaspoons lemon juice
1 piece fresh ginger, grated (approximately 2 cm)
2 cloves garlic, chopped
1 tablespoon olive oil

Method

1. Dry-roast the sesame seeds in a small pan over medium heat until golden.
2. Wash and trim the greens to pieces of similar length.
3. Mix the sesame oil, tamari, lemon juice, ginger and garlic in a small bowl.
4. Heat in a wok the olive oil until hot, add the broccolini and cook for approximately 1 minute.
5. Add the remaining greens and toss the dressing through at the same time.
6. Cook for a further 2 minutes.
7. Serve on a platter with sesame seeds sprinkled over the top.

Lentil Dhal *Serves 4*

It may seem like cheap peasant food, but you'll be surprised how enjoyable and satisfying dhal is if you haven't had it before. Lentils (pulses) are much easier to digest than legumes (beans) and, unlike beans, don't require any soaking.

Ingredients

1 tablespoon olive oil
1 onion, peeled and finely chopped
1 large red capsicum, finely chopped
2 cloves garlic, crushed
1 tablespoon fresh peeled and grated ginger
½ teaspoon ground ginger
1 teaspoon all spice
½ teaspoon chilli flakes
½ teaspoon ground cloves
1½ cups red lentils, rinsed and drained
2 fresh bay leaves
1 cup water
3 cups vegetable stock

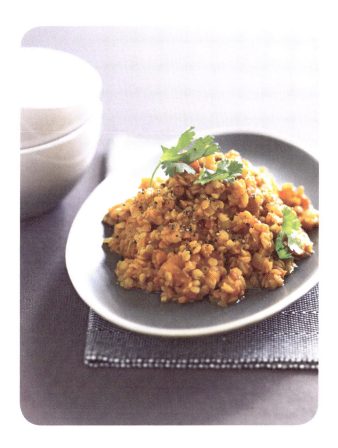

Method

1. Heat the olive oil in a medium-sized saucepan.
2. Add the onion, capsicum, garlic, fresh ginger and ground spices and sauté for 3–4 minutes.
3. Add the lentils, bay leaves, water and vegetable stock and bring to the boil.
4. Reduce the heat and simmer partially covered for 40 minutes until the lentils are tender and most of the liquid is absorbed.
5. Serve with cucumber, yoghurt and mint dip, steamed greens and a grain.

Note: To complete the protein and make all 8 essential amino acids, lentils should be served with a grain. Rice or chapattis are the traditional accompaniments to dhal. If you do want to use rice, use brown rice.

5-star performing foods—pearl barley

'Better than Mash' Barley and Bean Pot *Serves 4*

There are plenty of things to serve with a meal other than mashed potato and boiled rice. This barley and bean pot is delicious served with grilled lamb, chicken (see recipe for Barbecued Chicken and Preserved Lemon on page 192) or fish.

Ingredients

1 cup pearl barley
2 cups water
2 cups chicken stock
2 cups green beans, trimmed and cut in half lengthways

Method

1. Rinse the barley thoroughly in cold water.
2. In a medium-sized pan, add the barley, water and stock and bring to the boil. Reduce the heat and simmer uncovered for 40 minutes, stirring occasionally, until the grain is soft and most of the liquid has absorbed into the grain.
3. Add the beans and cook for a further 5 minutes.

5-star performing foods—sweet corn, olive oil

Barbecued Corn with Lemon Infused Olive Oil *Serves 4*

Flavoured olive oils are becoming increasingly popular and are available from most good delis. If you can't find any, simply combine fresh lemon juice with olive oil in the ratio of 1:3.

Ingredients

4 whole sweet corns cob with the husks on
2 tablespoons lemon infused olive oil
cracked black pepper

Method

1. Soak the cobs in water for about 5 minutes.
2. Lay the corn on an oiled hot plate and cook the cobs for 15–20 minutes, turning regularly to prevent the husks becoming too brown.
3. Strip back the husks, leaving them on the cob to be used as a handle. Drizzle with lemon infused olive oil, sprinkle with black pepper and serve.

Garlic and Chickpea Mash *Serves 4*

With a good food processor, you'll soon come to love using beans and chickpeas as a replacement for potato and rice. Here we mix chickpeas with roasted garlic to further pack it with nutritional punch.

Ingredients

½ bulb garlic (skin left on)
1 × 400 g can chickpeas, drained and rinsed
1 tablespoon olive oil
1 teaspoon chilli oil
½ cup finely chopped parsley
sea salt and black pepper

Method

1. Preheat the oven to 180°C.
2. Place the garlic on a small tray in the oven to roast for 25 minutes or until soft.
3. Peel the garlic and squeeze it into a food processor. Add the chickpeas and process for 1–2 minutes.
4. Add the oils and continue to process until smooth.
5. Stir through the chopped parsley and season to taste.
6. Serve warm under grilled lamb or as a spread in sandwiches.

Cracked Sweet and Sour Freekeh *Serves 4*

Forget the gloopy sauce used to make sweet and sour dishes in Chinese restaurants. The combination of prunes and preserved lemons is delicious with freekeh. This salad can be served as an accompaniment to barbecued chicken or roast duck.

Ingredients

1 cup cracked freekeh
8 pitted prunes, finely chopped
2 preserved lemons, flesh removed and discarded and skin finely chopped
1 cup continental parsley, finely chopped
cracked black pepper
a pinch sea salt

Method

1. Cook the freekeh as per instructions on the packet.
2. While still warm, combine with remaining ingredients and serve.

Spicy Red Cabbage with Cranberries *Serves 6*

Red cabbage and cranberries for a multitude of antioxidants, spices to boost the metabolism and aid digestion, and a wonderful fusion of flavours make this variation on a traditional German dish an excellent companion to turkey, duck or chicken.

Ingredients

1 tablespoon corn oil
1 Spanish (red) onion, finely chopped
2 cloves garlic, crushed
½ teaspoon cinnamon
½ teaspoon ground nutmeg
½ tablespoon grated fresh ginger
½ red cabbage, sliced thinly
1½ tablespoons apple cider vinegar
2 tablespoons apple concentrate
½ cup frozen cranberries

Method

1. Heat the oil in a heavy based pan.
2. Add the onion and garlic and sauté for 2 minutes.
3. Add the spices and cabbage, vinegar and apple concentrate and stir through.
4. Reduce the heat to low and cover the pan.
5. Cook for 20 minutes.
6. Add the cranberries, stir through and cook for a further 15 minutes.

Note: Cranberries are grown in North America and are only available frozen from the supermarket.

Brussels Sprouts with Roasted Pine Nut and Lemon Mustard Dressing *Serves 4*

Anyone who's eaten overcooked Brussels sprouts will never want to eat them again. Fear and loathing is the common complaint made against these poor misunderstood greens. Brussels sprouts must be cooked through—neither too crisp nor grey and mushy. Select them all of similar size and test them with a small sharp knife after 5 minutes and every minute thereafter.

Ingredients

24 Brussels sprouts, medium sized
¼ cup pine nuts
1½ tablespoons olive oil
juice of ½ lemon
1 teaspoon deseeded mustard
1 lemon, grated zest only

Method

1. Trim the Brussels sprouts and remove the outer leaves. Using a sharp knife, make a cross incision at the base of each sprout.
2. Dry-roast the pine nuts in a small frying pan over medium heat, taking care not to burn them.
3. Steam the sprouts for approximately 5–7 minutes, depending on their size. Drain thoroughly.
4. In a small saucepan, heat the olive oil, stir in the lemon juice, mustard and pine nuts.
5. Toss through the sprouts and serve immediately topped with grated lemon zest.

Dinner

Were we only to eat for health, we'd be best advised to eat the main meal of the day at lunchtime, with the smaller meal reserved for the end of the day. In doing so, the food would be well on its way to being digested before going to bed. Given, however, that the aim is to eat for health and pleasure, and most of us don't have a lifestyle to accommodate leisurely mid-day eating, the main meal of the day will invariably be served in the evening. Make an occasion of the main meal in the day. Sit down at the table, switch off the TV and take time to enjoy your food while relaxing with your family or friends. And, to ensure a good night's sleep, give yourself a few hours after eating before going to bed.

Meat

It's a personal choice whether to eat meat or not, but after reading Joanna's section I'm sure you'll agree there's no disputing its value in a healthy diet. The great thing these days is there are so many lean cuts of meat available. Bear in mind if you cook lean meat for too long it will turn out tough. Regardless it's always better to enjoy meat rare or medium rare as overcooked chargrilled meat produces carcinogens.

Chilli Beef and Beans *Serves 4*

An old favourite with students in the Northern Hemisphere on a tight budget who need to fill up, heat up and don't want to go to a lot of effort.

Commonly served with rice or on large baked potatoes, chilli beef and beans is better served with quinoa or with extra beans and a large salad.

Ingredients

1 tablespoon olive oil
1 large brown onion, peeled and finely chopped
2 cloves garlic, peeled and crushed
2 small red chillies, deseeded and finely chopped
350 g premium lean minced beef
1 × 400 g can whole tomatoes, chopped
1 tablespoon tomato paste
500 ml beef stock
1 green capsicum, finely diced
400 g can (or pre-cooked dried) kidney beans

Method

1. Pour oil into pan and sauté the onion and garlic for 3–4 minutes until soft.
2. Add the chilli and minced beef and cook gently until the beef is evenly browned.
3. Add the tomatoes, tomato paste, beef stock, capsicum and kidney beans and bring to the boil.
4. Reduce the heat to simmer, partially cover the pan and cook on the stove top for 45 minutes or until the liquid has reduced down to a thick sauce.

> **Tip:** *Chilli beef and beans is nice stuffed into halved red capsicums, covered in foil and baked in the oven for 20–25 minutes.*

Rolled Beef with Asparagus and Shallots *Makes 16 pieces, serves 4*

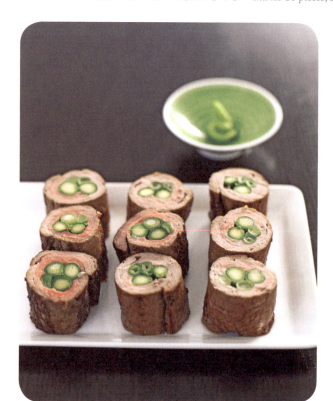

Combining asparagus and shallots, these pretty little rolls make an excellent main dish served with buckwheat noodles or brown sushi rice.

Ingredients

8 stalks asparagus

8 shallots

450 g of beef sirloin, beaten with a mallet into 4 very thin sheets

2 tablespoons grapeseed oil

50 ml sake

½ tablespoon rice syrup

1½ tablespoons mirin

2 tablespoons salt-reduced soy sauce

wasabi paste, to serve

Note: Sake is an alcoholic Japanese rice wine available from Asian stores. While there are some reports suggesting sake has numerous health benefits, it, like all other alcoholic beverages, should be consumed in moderation. It also contains no sulphites—the chemicals found in white wine and dried fruit that can cause asthma-like symptoms in some. When cooking with alcohol, the alcohol content is burned off.

Method

1. Break the ends off the asparagus, cut in half.
2. Trim the shallots at the roots and cut them to the length of the asparagus.
3. Place the asparagus and shallots in a steamer for 2–3 minutes until the asparagus is tender.
4. Refresh in cold water.
5. Spread beef slices on a board, and lay two asparagus and shallot pieces onto each piece of meat.
6. Roll the beef around the vegetables and trim the ends.
7. Heat oil in a frying pan and brown the rolls.
8. Remove from the pan and set aside.
9. Combine the sake, rice syrup, mirin and soy sauce in the frying pan and cook for 5–6 minutes to reduce.
10. Return the beef rolls to the pan and toss around to coat with the sauce.
11. Cut the rolls into pieces approx 2½ cm wide and arrange in a serving dish.
12. Serve with wasabi paste.

Eye Fillet with Salsa Verde *Serves 4*

The translation of salsa verde is green sauce, which is probably why we've adopted the Italian name. It has a strong taste and is delicious on full-flavoured fish like mackerel and tuna as well as red meat.

Ingredients

4 eye fillets of beef (approximately 200 g each)

Salsa verde

1 cup curly leaf parsley
1 cup flat leaf parsley
2 cloves garlic, crushed
¼ cup capers, rinsed and drained
2 teaspoons creamed horseradish
juice of 1 large lemon
¼ cup olive oil
ground black pepper

Method

1. To make the salsa verde, place the parsley, garlic, capers, horseradish and lemon in a food processor and process until combined.
2. Slowly add the olive oil and process until the sauce has a consistent texture. Season with black pepper.
3. Oil the steaks with a brush of olive oil and set aside.
4. Heat a grill pan and cook the steaks for 3–5 minutes on each side depending on how you like your steak cooked.
5. Serve with the salsa verde on top.

Marinated Lamb and Vegetable Kebabs *Serves 4*

Even though there is less saturated fat on trimmed cuts of meat, there is and never has been any fibre. Are the high incidents of colon cancer a result of too much meat or not enough vegetables? There is much research to suggest the latter. So, whenever you have a meat dish, do as we have done in this dish and incorporate several extra veggies.

Ingredients

¼ cup olive oil
1 tablespoon honey
2 cloves garlic
juice of 1 large lemon
1 tablespoon chopped mint,
1 tablespoon chopped rosemary leaves
1 red chilli, finely chopped
black pepper, to season
250 gm button mushrooms, cleaned
1 Spanish (red) onion, chopped into wedges
3 baby eggplant, chopped into 2 cm pieces
3 zucchini, chopped into 2 cm pieces
500 g trim lamb, diced

Method

1. Combine the olive oil with the honey, garlic, lemon juice, herbs, chilli and pepper in a small bowl.
2. Pour the marinade over the lamb and set aside to marinate for at least 30 minutes.
3. Thread the lamb and vegetables onto pre-soaked bamboo skewers, reserving the marinade to baste.
4. Seal the meat under a hot grill or on a hotplate for 3–4 minutes, turning and basting with reserved marinade occasionally.
5. Reduce the heat and cook for a further 3–4 minutes for medium or 4–5 minutes for well done.

Healthy Harira *Serves 4*

This delicious Moroccan lamb dish has the double bonus of two fabulous carbs—barley and lentils. It makes a hearty mid-week meal in winter and tastes even better the day after making.

Ingredients

1 tablespoon olive oil
250 gm lean lamb, cut into cubes
1 brown onion, peeled and chopped
1 pinch saffron threads
½ teaspoon cinnamon
½ teaspoon ground turmeric
¾ teaspoon ground ginger
2 tablespoons pearl barley
1½ litres vegetable stock
½ cup green lentils
1 x 800 g can tomatoes
1 tablespoon tomato paste (no sugar or salt added)
1 red capsicum, deseeded and chopped
1 bunch coriander leaves, roughly chopped
juice of 1 lemon
sea salt and black pepper

Method

1. Heat the oil in a large heavy-based pan, add the lamb and fry for about 2 minutes until the pieces are brown.
2. Add the onion and spices and cook until the onion is soft.
3. Add the barley and stock and bring to the boil.
4. Reduce to simmer and cook for 30 minutes.
5. Add the lentils, tomatoes, tomato paste and capsicum and cook for a further 30 minutes until the lentils are tender.
6. Stir in the coriander and lemon juice just before serving and season to taste.

Kangaroo Fillets with Macadamia and Plum Sauce *Serves 4*

What could be more Australian—kangaroo with macadamias! The strong flavour of the meat offset against the plum and macadamia sauce is delicious and, of course, beautiful served with a fresh green salad.

Ingredients

3 medium plums, pitted and cut into small cubes
½ tablespoon apple concentrate
½ tablespoon finely grated fresh ginger
1 tablespoon water
2 tablespoons chopped mint
½ teaspoon tamari
½ teaspoon lemon juice
600 g kangaroo fillets
olive oil
black pepper
1 tablespoon unsalted macadamias, lightly toasted and chopped

Method

1. Place the chopped plums in a small pan with the apple concentrate, ginger and water. Bring to the boil, cover and reduce heat and simmer until the water has been absorbed and the plum resembles plum jam. Remove from the heat and set aside to cool.
2. Once the sauce has cooled a little, add mint, tamari and lemon juice.
3. Preheat the oven to 150°C. Slice kangaroo fillets into approximately 125 g portions and, using a meat mallet, gently flatten the fillets out.
4. Heat the oil in the pan, seal kangaroo fillets on both sides, season with pepper and place in warm oven for 10 minutes and allow to finish cooking while still being rare in the centre.
5. Serve the plum sauce over the kangaroo fillets with the macadamias over the top. Serve with a green salad.

Note: Kangaroo is extremely lean and will become very tough if overcooked. It should be served pink and rare.

Chargrilled Kangaroo Steaks with Hummus, Silverbeet, and Beetroot and Apple Relish *Serves 4*

With its strong flavour, this beetroot and apple relish is delicious with gamey meats such as kangaroo. The relish recipe makes double quantities to store in the fridge and use again. It's also delicious with grilled veggies and goat cheese.

Ingredients

4 kangaroo steaks (approximately 150 g each)

1 tablespoon olive oil

1 bunch silverbeet, stalks removed and trimmed

¾ cup hummus

4 tablespoons beetroot and apple relish, see recipe below

Note: When buying hummus, always check the ingredient list and buy a brand free of any artificial preservatives and other additives.

Beetroot and Apple Relish

1 tablespoon safflower oil

2 Spanish (red) onions, peeled and finely chopped

4 medium beetroots, peeled and chopped into cubes approximately 1 cm

2 green apples, peeled, cored and finely chopped

¾ cup white wine vinegar

2 tablespoons apple concentrate

¼ teaspoon ground cloves

½ cup boiling water

Note: To sterilise glass jars, wash thoroughly in hot soapy water and rinse thoroughly. Place the jars on a baking tray in the oven preheated to 120°C for 20 minutes.

Method

1. To make the relish, place all the ingredients in a heavy-based pan and slowly bring to the boil.
2. Reduce to simmer, cover and cook for approximately 45 minutes until the liquid has absorbed and the ingredients are soft and pulpy.
3. Set aside to cool before transferring to a sterilised storage jar.
4. Preheat the oven to 180°C.
5. Brush the steaks with olive oil and sear on a grill pan on both sides for 2 minutes.
6. Transfer to a baking tray and place in the oven to cook through for a further 10 minutes.
7. Bring a large pan of water to boil and blanch the silverbeet for 2 minutes. Drain thoroughly and squeeze excess moisture from it.
8. Serve the kangaroo on a bed of silverbeet with accompanying hummus and beetroot relish

Grilled Chicken with Smoked Paprika, Chilli and Capsicum Sauce *Serves 4*

The sauce in this dish can be used in any variety of ways other than as we have done here with grilled chicken. It's delicious over grilled lamb, lentil burgers and even as a dip with vegetable crudités.

Ingredients

1 red capsicum
2 large red chilli peppers
4 small organic chicken breasts
olive oil
1 small red chilli, deseeded and finely chopped
juice of ½ lemon
½ teaspoon smoked paprika
pinch sea salt

Method

1. Preheat the oven to 180°C.
2. Grill the capsicum and chilli peppers until they have blackened all over.
3. Remove from the grill and place them in a plastic bag to cool.
4. Brush the chicken with olive oil and chargrill on each side for 2–3 minutes.
5. Transfer to a baking tray and place in the oven to cook through for 15 minutes.
6. Peel the skin from the capsicum and peppers and place in a food processor.
7. Add the chilli, lemon juice, paprika and seasoning and process until it's smooth
8. Serve over grilled chicken with steamed greens.

Chicken and Tomato Bake *Serves 4*

We've snuck in a little grated Parmesan to give the quinoa a slight golden crust and sharper flavour. Although a saturated fat, a little goes a long way when it's grated.

Ingredients

500 g organic chicken breasts
1½ cups tomato and basil sauce (see recipe, page 173)
1 cup quinoa
2 cups water
¼ cup grated Parmesan
1 bunch English spinach

Method

1. Preheat oven to 180°C.
2. Cut the chicken into strips approximately 1 cm thick.
3. Arrange them in a baking dish and cover with a layer of tomato and basil sauce. Cover with foil and bake for 20–25 minutes.
4. Add the quinoa to the water and bring to the boil.
5. Cover the pan and reduce to simmer for 15 minutes until the water is completely absorbed and the quinoa is soft.
6. Stir the Parmesan through the quinoa.
7. Top the chicken and tomato and basil sauce with the quinoa and Parmesan mix, and return to the oven for a further 10 minutes.
8. Steam the English spinach for 3 minutes.
9. Remove chicken bake from the oven and serve immediately with the spinach.

Barbecued Chicken with Preserved Lemon *Serves 4*

Preserved lemon is made with lemon juice and a lot of salt, which of course is not a big plus when it comes to good health. If, however, your diet is relatively free of packaged food products and you don't add salt to your food, automatically you are eating less salt than the average person. That's my justification anyway to include a small amount of this wonderful condiment in your cooking. When using preserved lemons, discard the fleshy pulp and use the peel only.

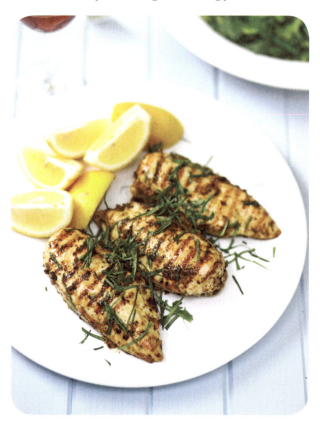

Ingredients

4 pieces preserved lemon
2 tablespoons lemon juice
2 cloves garlic
1 teaspoon ground cumin
1 teaspoon sweet paprika
⅓ cup olive oil
cracked black pepper
¼ bunch coriander leaves, roughly chopped
2 coriander roots, washed
4 organic chicken breasts

Method

1. Remove the pulp from the preserved lemon and add the rind to a food processor with the lemon juice, garlic, cumin, paprika, oil, pepper, coriander leaves and roots and process until smooth.
2. Wipe the chicken breasts with damp paper towel to clean and smear the marinade over each of them.
3. Set aside to marinate in the refrigerator for 1–2 hours.
4. Preheat barbecue grill.
5. Cook chicken on the barbecue for approximately 7 minutes each side turning once.

Fish

Fish is one of the healthiest sources of protein available. It's rich in omega-3 fatty acids, low in saturated fat, and is easy to prepare and cook. Buy it fresh and cook on the day of buying and, where possible, buy Australian rather than imported. Approximately three-quarters of the world's oceans are fished up to their limits with as much as 90 per cent of the large predatory fish such as bluefin tuna, shark and swordfish lost. These fish also have a higher concentration of mercury and are best avoided (see page 90 for more information), to preserve both our ecosystem and our health.

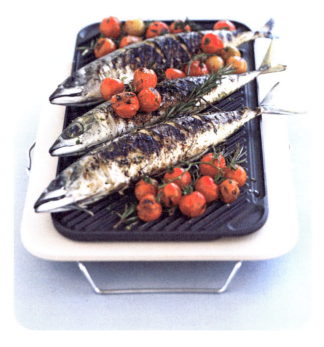

Mediterranean Mackerel with Basil and Rocket Pesto. Refer to page 196

5-star performing foods—garlic, olive oil, pearl barley, salmon, lime, onion, peas

Barley and Pea Risotto with Chargrilled Salmon *Serves 4*

While it doesn't have the creamy consistency of rice risotto, this barley risotto is just as comforting with many more health benefits. Once you get used to making risotto with barley, there's no going back.

Ingredients

2 large cloves garlic, crushed
1 tablespoon olive oil
3 cups fish stock
1 cup pearl barley, rinsed
4 salmon fillets, skin left on
olive oil, extra
juice of 1 lime
freshly ground black pepper
2 shallots, finely chopped
1 cup fresh shelled peas
½ cup chopped chervil

Method

1. Preheat the oven to 180°C.
2. Sauté the garlic and olive oil in a heavy-based oven-proof dish for 2 minutes. Add the fish stock and gently bring it to the boil.
3. Add the barley, cover the pan with a lid and transfer to the middle shelf of the oven for 50 minutes.
4. After the barley has been cooking for approximately 40 minutes, brush the salmon fillets with olive oil, lime juice and season with black pepper.
5. Heat an oiled grill pan and sear the salmon on the skin side for 2 minutes. Turn and sear on the other side for another minute. Remove from the heat and set aside.
6. Remove the barley risotto from the oven, add the shallots and peas, then lay the fish on top.
7. Return to the oven for 10 minutes.
8. Remove from the oven, sprinkle the chervil on top and serve with a green salad.

Grilled Snapper Fillet with Bulgur, Parsley and Roasted Almonds *Serves 4*

Served with a chilli and capsicum sauce (see page 190), this meal tastes and looks stunning.

Ingredients

1 cup bulgur
2 cups water
¼ cup almonds, dry-roasted in a pan and roughly chopped
½ cup continental parsley, chopped
4 snapper fillets
olive oil for brushing
1 tablespoon lemon juice
cracked black pepper

Method

1. Preheat the oven to 200°C.
2. Soak the bulgur in 2 cups boiling water for 30 minutes.
3. Squeeze any excess moisture from the soaked bulgur and mix through the roast almonds and chopped parsley.
4. Brush the snapper with a little olive oil, lemon juice and black pepper and grill for 5 minutes each side.
5. Serve the snapper over the bulgur with chilli and capsicum sauce and a green salad.

Mediterranean Mackerel with Basil and Rocket Pesto *Serves 4*

A casual barbecue with fresh mackerel can look impressive yet be extremely economical. The freshest mackerel is required here and, for the brave, better to cut and clean it yourself. The less handling prior to cooking, the better.

Ingredients

4 × 1 kg whole Slimy mackerel (cleaned and gutted)
350 g vine-ripened cherry tomatoes
4 sprigs thyme
4 sprigs rosemary

Basil and Rocket Pesto

¼ bunch basil
¼ bunch rocket leaves
zest and juice of 1 lemon
2 cloves garlic, crushed
¼ cup extra virgin olive oil
cracked black pepper

Method

1. Preheat a grill or barbecue and brush with oil.
2. To make the pesto, add the basil, rocket, lemon juice and zest, garlic, oil and seasoning to a blender and blend until all the ingredients are well combined.
3. Score the mackerel along the sides at the thickest parts of its body and rub in the basil and rocket pesto both inside and out.
4. Place the fish on the grill and place the herbs and tomatoes on the plate.
5. Cook fish for 25–30 minutes turning once after 15 minutes. Turn herbs and tomatoes regularly to prevent charring.
6. Serve with a fresh green salad.

Mackerel

Mackerel is available canned, smoked and of course fresh. Its strong flavour may put some reluctant fish-eaters off but, for those of you who love fish, it's an excellent fish to combine with other interesting full flavours. It's one of the best fish for omega-3 fatty acids, containing more than 100 milligrams per 100 gram.

There are a number of species of mackerel, distinguished mainly by their size. The largest and best known is the Spanish mackerel, usually sold in cutlets. If you are concerned about mercury, the smaller varieties, including Slimy and Blue, are a better option.

All fish is better fresh, but none more so than mackerel. The fish must be sleek, dark, glossy and firm. If it bends when held by the head and tail, don't buy it.

Baked Ling with Eggplant, Capsicum and Lima Beans *Serves 4*

Ling is a firm-fleshed white fish. If unavailable, try blue-eye cod or snapper.

Ingredients

¼ cup olive oil
2 medium eggplant, cut into cubes approximately 3 cm
3 large vine ripened tomatoes, diced
2 red capsicums cut into strips
1 small bird's eye chilli
4 cloves garlic, crushed
4 ling fillets
olive oil, to brush fish
lemon juice, to brush fish
1 x can lima beans, drained
cracked black pepper
sea salt

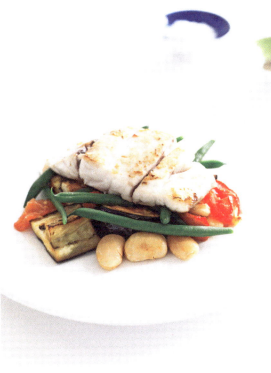

Method

1. Preheat oven to 180°C.
2. Heat the oil in a baking tray until hot. Remove from the oven and add the eggplant, tomato, capsicum, chilli and garlic.
3. Toss through so the olive oil is covering all the vegetables and return to the oven to cook for 10 minutes.
4. While the veggies are cooking, brush the ling with a little olive oil and lemon juice and sear in a non-stick pan for 1–2 minutes on each side. Then, lay the fish on a separate tray lined with baking paper and cook for a further 10 minutes in the oven.
5. Remove the veggies from the oven, add the lima beans and gently toss through. Season with salt and pepper.
6. Place the veggie mixture on serving plates. Top with the cooked ling. Serve with steamed greens.

Ruby Red Ocean Trout *Serves 4*

The combination of grapefruit and tomatoes with the trout is superb and looks particularly magnificent served with silverbeet and olive oil.

Ingredients

2 ruby red grapefruit, segmented
½ cup mint
4 roma tomatoes, deseeded
1 tablespoon extra virgin olive oil
1 clove garlic, crushed
cracked black pepper
4 ocean trout fillets

Method

1. Slice between the membranes of the ruby red grapefruits to remove the pith.
2. Finely slice the mint and dice the ripe roma tomatoes.
3. Warm the olive oil in a pan, add the garlic, tomatoes and cracked pepper and simmer for 5 minutes.
4. Add the mint and grapefruit segments and continue to simmer with the juice from the grapefruit.
5. While the sauce is cooking, grill the trout for approximately 3–5 minutes on each side depending on how you like it cooked.
6. Lay the vegetable and grapefruit mix on serving plates and arrange the cooked trout on top.

Grapefruit

In Oriental medicine the grapefruit is used to treat alcohol intoxication, poor digestion and belching!.

Grilled Blue-Eye Cod with Sage, Lentils and Roast Capsicum *Serves 2*

Lentils combined with preserved limes and roast capsicum make a delicious base to this easy fish dish.

Ingredients

2 blue-eye cod fillets (approximately 150 g each)
½ tablespoon olive oil
juice of ½ lemon
1 tablespoon olive oil, extra
1 tablespoon capers, rinsed and drained
½ bunch sage leaves
1 x can lentils, drained and rinsed
2 preserved limes, flesh scraped and discarded, rind finely chopped
1 ready-prepared roast capsicum, sliced

Method

1. Preheat the oven to 180°C.
2. Wipe the fish with a damp cloth.
3. Make a few incisions across the thickest part of the fillets and brush with ½ tablespoon olive oil and lemon juice.
4. Heat the extra olive oil until hot but not smoking and add the capers and sage leaves. Cook until they're crispy.
5. Remove from the oil and lay them out on absorbent paper towel to drain them of excess oil.
6. Heat a grill pan and sear the fish for 2 minutes on each side, then transfer the fish to a baking tray and cook in the oven for 15–20 minutes to cook through.
7. While the fish is cooking, heat the lentils in a pan and stir through the preserved limes and capsicum.
8. When the fish is cooked, sprinkle the capers and sage through the lentils.
9. Serve fish on top of the lentils with an accompanying green salad.

Poached Ocean Trout with Green Tea Salsa *Serves 4*

It's not often you can serve up a meal with a real point of difference, as you can with this dish. The green tea combined in a salsa and served with trout poached in green tea is absolutely delicious and very different—not forgetting the numerous health benefits.

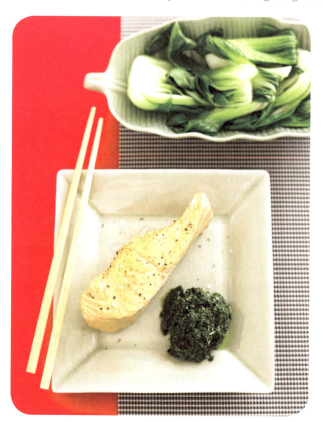

Ingredients

4 tablespoons sencha tea
6 cups boiling water
4 skinless trout fillets
1 bunch coriander leaves
3 coriander roots, scraped clean
½ cup flat leaf parsley
¼ cup extra virgin camellia tea oil
1 tablespoon green tea leaves
juice of 1 lime
3 anchovy fillets, drained of oil
black pepper
1 bunch bok choy

Note: Sencha is loose leaf Japanese green tea with a stronger flavour than Chinese green teas. It can be purchased from most Asian grocers.

Method

1. Place the sencha tea leaves in a pan with the water and steep for 5 minutes. Strain the tea of leaves and return to the pan.
2. Place the trout fillets into the pan, making sure they are completely covered in tea and, over a moderate heat, bring the tea back to the boil. As soon as the tea starts to boil, turn off the heat and cover the pan. Leave the trout to sit in the water for approximately 1 hour.
3. Place the coriander leaves and roots, parsley, camellia tea oil, green tea, lime juice, anchovies and black pepper in a food processor and process until smooth.
4. Strain the trout and serve with the salsa on top accompanied with steamed bok choy.

Chargrilled Salmon with Asparagus, Lemon and Anchovy *Serves 4*

In less than 30 minutes you can be sitting down to this extremely healthy meal which tastes as good as any dish served in a great restaurant.

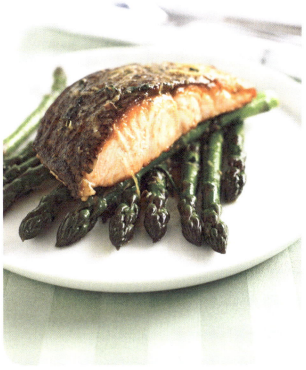

Ingredients

4 salmon fillets
olive oil for brushing fish
3 bunches asparagus
⅓ cup cold pressed extra virgin olive oil
8 anchovies
½ cup chopped flat leaf parsley
2 tablespoons lemon juice and zest of 1 lemon
black pepper

Method

1. Preheat the oven to 180°C.
2. Wipe the salmon fillets clean with damp paper towel and brush lightly with olive oil. Heat a grill pan and sear the salmon for approximately 2 minutes on each side.
3. Transfer to a baking tray and place in the oven for 10–15 minutes depending on how you like it cooked.
4. Place the asparagus spears in a pan with just enough boiling water to cover them. Cook for 2 minutes until they are tender but still crisp. Drain, remove asparagus and keep warm.
5. Heat the olive oil in the same pan.
6. Drain and blot the anchovies of oil before mashing them with a fork.
7. Add the anchovy paste to the olive oil.
8. Return the asparagus to the pan with the parsley and spoon the anchovy and oil over the spears.
9. Add the lemon juice and black pepper and serve under the salmon steaks.

Note: *After eating asparagus, you may notice a strong odour in your urine. This is totally harmless and is thought to result from a breakdown product produced during metabolism of the amino acid asparagine found in asparagus. This amino acid was first isolated from asparagus and hence its name! Asparagine is a non-essential amino acid, meaning that we can make it in the body from other amino acids. It plays an important role in the nervous system as well as in the production of other amino acids.*

Baked Kingfish and Mushrooms *Serves 4*

The 'freedom with fish club' is one that you'll automatically join when you realise there are few boundaries when serving fish. With the technique of cooking fish down pat, you will quickly learn that, like meat, it can be combined with any vegetable, served with a multitude of sauces and laid on top of anything you would lay a piece of steak on. Here we combine the delicate flavours of various mushrooms with one of our favourite fish, kingfish.

Ingredients

¼ cup olive oil
2 cloves garlic, crushed
400 g mixed mushrooms, chopped (brown, shiitake, oyster, button)
1 cup fish stock
pinch sea salt
cracked black pepper
4 kingfish fillets
olive oil for brushing fish
½ bunch flat leaf parsley

Method

1. Preheat the oven to 200°C.
2. Heat the oil in a pan and add garlic and mushrooms. Cook over a medium heat for about 4 minutes.
3. Add the stock and the seasoning, simmer for a further 4 minutes and set aside.
4. Brush the kingfish fillets with olive oil. Heat a non-stick pan and sear the fish (skin side first) for 1 minute. Turn it over and sear the other side for 30 seconds.
5. Transfer the fish to a baking tray and place in the oven for 3–4 minutes.
6. Gently reheat the mushrooms and add the parsley.
7. Serve the fish on top of a bed of mushrooms and accompany the dish with some lightly steamed English spinach.

Note: Like tuna, kingfish can easily turn from a succulent moist fish to bone dry when cooked. Take care not to overcook it.

Kingfish with Pine Nuts and Cucumber and Lemon Salsa *Serves 4*

Ingredients

½ cup pine nuts

2 tablespoons fresh rosemary leaves

4 kingfish fillets (approximately 150 g each)

Salsa

2 Lebanese cucumbers

juice of 1 lemon

2 segments of preserved lemon peel, finely chopped

1 tablespoon chopped mint

Method

1. To make the salsa, slice the cucumber thinly using a potato peeler.
2. Place the slices in a non-reactive bowl and add the lemon juice, preserved lemon and mint. Mix it all together and rest a plate over the surface to weigh the ingredients down.
3. Chill in the refrigerator for 2–3 hours.
4. To prepare the remainder of the dish, grind the pine nuts and rosemary together in a spice grinder.
5. Press the mixture over each side of the kingfish with the flat blade of a knife. Cover the grill plate with silver foil and grill the fish over a moderate heat for 4 minutes each side, taking care not to burn the pine nuts.
6. Serve with cucumber and lemon salsa and steamed spinach.

Vegetarian

Not so many years ago, a meal devoid of meat was incomplete and only enjoyed by unshaven weirdos! Fortunately, this closed mentality is now a thing of the past as the mainstream finally recognises that many vegetarian dishes are more creative, beautiful and delicious than those using meat, poultry or fish can ever be.

5-star performing foods—olive oil, garlic, mushrooms, lentils

Spring Veggie Pie *Serves 6*

There's something so fulfilling about making a pie from scratch and so satisfying to sit down to eat. This rustic pie takes a little time but is very easy and enjoyable to make—particularly when it's designed to look imperfect! The true perfectionists may want to cook their own lentils, but canned work just as well and remove a step from this labour of love.

Poppy Seed Pastry

1 cup wholemeal spelt flour

¾ cup white spelt flour

pinch sea salt

1 tablespoon poppy seeds

⅓ cup omega spread (see notes)

¼ cup iced cold water

Filling

1 tablespoon olive oil

250 g pumpkin, peeled

3 cloves garlic

1 tablespoon rosemary

250 g mushrooms

200 g green beans, trimmed and cut into pieces approximately 3 cm long

1 × 400 g can lentils, drained and rinsed

2 tablespoons shiro miso

⅓ cup water

Notes: Frozen, pre rolled pastry is likely to contain trans fats, known to reduce levels of protective (HDL) cholesterol while increasing levels of harmful (LDL) cholesterol.

Omega spread is available from health food stores and is made from a blend of omega-3 and omega-6 fatty acids using a cold process which does not involve hydrogenation. It contains no trans fats or cholesterol.

Method

1. To make the pastry, place the flours, seasoning, omega spread and poppy seeds in a food processor.
2. Process until well combined.
3. Slowly add the iced water while the processor is still on until the dough is stiff enough to form a ball.
4. Place the dough in the refrigerator for 20–25 minutes.
5. Preheat the oven to 180°C.
6. To make the filling, heat the olive oil in a baking tray and, once hot, add the pumpkin, garlic, rosemary and mushrooms. Toss through and place in the oven to roast for 15–20 minutes.
7. Steam the green beans for 4 minutes then drain and refresh in cold water.
8. Mix the roasted veggies, lentils and beans together and set aside to cool.
9. Mix the shiro miso with water to a smooth paste and combine in the bowl with the lentils roast veggies and beans.
10. Roll the pastry out and place on a pizza stone or lined baking tray.
11. Fill the middle of the pastry with the lentils and veggies then fold it up and over the edges to form a rustic looking pie.
12. Bake in the oven for 20–25 minutes.

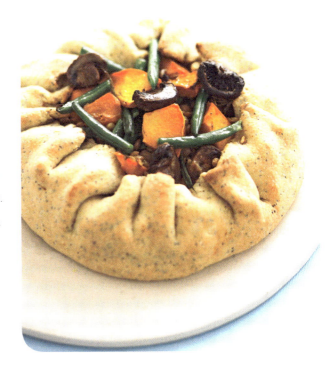

Sautéed Silverbeet, Olive and Fennel Pasta *Serves 4*

There are some things you should have in the refrigerator and pantry at all times. A good quality Parmesan (a little of it goes a long way so don't worry about the fat content), some kalamata olives, olive oil, wholemeal pasta and garlic. A quick dash to the shops to grab a bunch of spinach and fennel bulb and this mid-week dish can be on the table in minutes.

Ingredients

500 g wholemeal pasta
1 bunch silverbeet, washed and trimmed
1 tablespoon olive oil
2 cloves garlic, finely sliced
1 fennel bulb, thinly sliced
⅓ cup kalamata olives
2 tablespoons grated Parmesan
balck pepper

Method

1 Cook the pasta in plenty of boiling water for approx 15–20 minutes until it's soft but retains 'bite'.

2 Cook the silverbeet for 1 minute in plenty of boiling water. Drain thoroughly. Heat the olive oil in a large pan and cook the garlic until golden.

3 Add the fennel and cook for a further 3–5 minutes. Toss through the silverbeet and cook for a further 2 minutes. Remove from the heat and add the olives.

4 Serve the silverbeet mixture over the pasta. Top with a small amount of grated Parmesan and black pepper.

Silverbeet, Pumpkin and Pine Nut Roll *Serves 4*

This dish looks far more complicated than it actually is and tastes really delicious.

Ingredients

1 bunch silverbeet, washed and stalks removed
½ teaspoon nutmeg
sea salt and pepper
2–3 cups pumpkin, peeled and cut into chunks
6 egg whites
100 g soft goat's cheese
1 tablespoon pine nuts, roasted

Method

1. Preheat the oven to 180°C.
2. Cook the silverbeet in boiling water for 2 minutes. Plunge into cold water and squeeze dry.
3. Blend the silverbeet in a food processor with nutmeg and seasoning.
4. Brush the pumpkin with a little olive oil and sprinkle with a little sea salt and pepper and place on a baking tray. Place in the oven to bake for 20 minutes.
5. Beat the egg whites until stiff peaks form.
6. Gently fold the silverbeet through the egg whites, taking care not to over-beat them.
7. Line a baking sheet with baking paper and spread the egg white mixture over the tray. Place in the oven to cook for 10 minutes until it's cooked through but still soft and springy. Remove from oven and ease gently from the tray with a flat knife and spatula and lay it out on a clean tea towel.
8. Spread the goat's cheese over the egg white base and sprinkle the pine nuts on top.
9. Lay the roast pumpkin over the top of the pine nuts mashing it down gently with a fork.
10. Using the tea towel to guide you, roll it up and serve with a fresh green salad.

Green Tea Barley Risotto with Mushrooms and Asparagus *Serves 4*

Genmaicha is a Japanese green tea blended with popped and toasted brown rice. It's available from most Asian grocers and is popular with many who don't like the strong flavour of green tea. Used in this barley risotto, it makes a delicious nutty and nourishing low-GI meal the whole family will enjoy. To boost protein, serve the risotto under a piece of white fish steamed in ginger and light soy sauce.

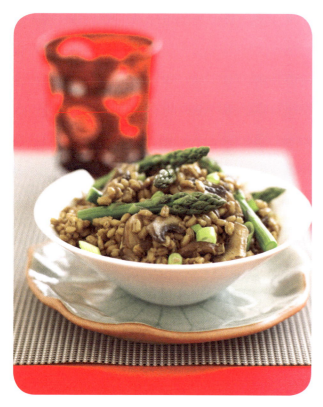

Ingredients

3 tablespoons camellia tea oil
200 g brown mushrooms, finely sliced
100 g shiitake mushrooms, finely sliced
2 cloves garlic, crushed
½ tablespoon grated fresh ginger
1 cup pearl barley
2½ cups genmaicha tea, strained
1 tablespoon tamari
10 stalks asparagus, trimmed and cut in half
5 shallots, finely sliced
2 limes

Method

1. Heat the camellia tea oil in a heavy-based pan. Sauté the mushrooms with the garlic and ginger for approximately 5 minutes.
2. Add the barley and stir around to coat the grains with oil.
3. Add the genmaicha and tamari and slowly bring to the boil.
4. Reduce to simmer, stir and cover the pan to cook for 1 hour. Check occasionally that the grain is not sticking to the bottom of the pan and add a little extra genmaicha if necessary.
5. Add the asparagus and shallots in the final 2 minutes of cooking
6. Serve with sliced fresh limes to sprinkle over the risotto.

Tofu, Broccoli and Sesame Stir-fry *Serves 2*

Ingredients

375 g organic firm tofu (cut into cubes)
1 tablespoon sesame oil
1 tablespoon olive oil
1 red capsicum, cut into strips
1 large red chilli, cut into fine strips
400 g broccoli (cut into small florets)
1 tablespoon sesame seeds

Tip: *The trick to giving tofu taste is to make it more porous before marinating it. This can be achieved either by boiling it first or freezing and defrosting it before you pour over the marinade.*

Sesame Sauce

2 tablespoons unhulled tahini
1 tablespoon mirin
1 tablespoon salt-reduced tamari
juice of ¼ lemon
juice of a 2 cm piece of grated ginger root
water

Method

1. To make the sesame sauce, mix the tahini together with the mirin, tamari, lemon juice and ginger juice. Add water until it reaches a smooth consistency (close to pouring cream).
2. To make the remainder of the dish, bring a medium-sized pan of water to the boil. Add the tofu cubes and return to the boil. Boil until the tofu cubes float to the surface of the water. Drain and blot dry.
3. Heat the sesame oil in a wok and stir-fry the tofu until it becomes slightly golden. Set aside to keep warm.
4. Heat the olive oil and stir-fry the capsicum and chilli for 2 minutes.
5. Add the broccoli florets and cook for a further 3 minutes, adding a little water if required.
6. Remove from the heat. Stir through the tofu and the sesame seeds. Drizzle with the sesame sauce or serve as a dipping sauce on the side.

Note: if you don't have a gas oven, it may be worth investing in an electric wok. Electric stoves can't heat woks to high enough temperatures for stir-frying.

Silverbeet, Ricotta and Vegetable Frittata *Serves 4–6*

Perhaps it's because they're so readily available, eggs don't generally excite the masses. But anyone who regularly makes frittatas will know, they are enjoyed by everyone when placed in front of them.

Ingredients

2 capsicums
1 onion, finely sliced
1 teaspoon olive oil
1 bunch silverbeet, stalks removed and cut into small pieces
250 g low-fat ricotta
¼ cup pickled gherkins, chopped finely
sea salt and cracked pepper
6 free range eggs

Method

1. Preheat the oven to 180°C.
2. Roast the capsicums in the oven until the skin is burnt and blistered. Set aside in a plastic bag until cool enough to remove the skin and seeds.
3. While the capsicum is roasting, fry the onion in the olive oil until golden and slightly crispy (approximately 10 minutes).
4. Blanch the silverbeet in boiling water for 2 minutes, drain and squeeze any excess moisture from it and set aside. Combine the silverbeet with the ricotta and gherkins, season with black pepper and a pinch of sea salt.
5. Separate the egg whites and beat until they form stiff peaks. Beat the egg yolks in a separate bowl then fold them into the egg white mixture.
6. Lightly grease a 2 litre oven-proof casserole dish with olive oil. Pour ½ the egg mixture into the bottom of the casserole then layer the onions and capsicum over the surface. Spread the silverbeet and ricotta mixture and then top with the remaining egg.
7. Cook in the centre of the oven for 20–25 minutes or until set. Serve with a green salad.

Sweet Things

We all enjoy a sweet treat now and again and there are ways of indulging your senses without too many liabilities. Making your own treats gets you half way there as you can ensure good quality ingredients without added undesirable extras. Here's a few of our favourites incorporating many of our 5-star performing foods.

5-star performing foods—ginger, hazelnuts, almonds, rolled oats, sunflower seeds, pepitas, sesame seeds

Rhubarb and Ginger Nut Crumble *Serves 6*

You could replace the rhubarb with pears, raspberries or any other fruit in season with this crumble topping. The topping is much healthier than the traditional crumble made from flour, sugar and butter—and far tastier! Dry-roast the nuts and seeds in a pan over medium heat until they are toasty but be careful not to burn them.

Ingredients

1 bunch rhubarb, trimmed
½ cup apple juice concentrate
1 teaspoon grated fresh ginger
¼ cup hazelnuts, dry-roasted
¼ cup almonds, dry-roasted
½ cup rolled oats, dry-roasted

¼ cup sunflower seeds, dry-roasted
¼ cup pepitas (pumpkin seeds), dry-roasted
1 tablespoon sesame seeds, dry-roasted
½ cup barley malt
1 tablespoon almond oil
¼ teaspoon ground cinnamon

Method

1. Preheat the oven to 160°C.
2. Wash the rhubarb but don't dry it, and cut into pieces about 2.5 cm long.
3. Put rhubarb in a pan over low heat, add the apple concentrate and ginger and cover. The rhubarb will slowly stew in the steam and its own juices.
4. Remove from the heat when the rhubarb is tender but still retains its shape—about 5–10 minutes. Divide rhubarb among 6 individual ramekins and set aside.
5. Coarsely chop the roasted nuts and mix with the oats and seeds.
6. Melt the barley malt in a saucepan with the almond oil and cinnamon and mix with a wooden spoon. Pour the oil and malt mixture over the nut mix and stir until thoroughly combined.
7. Spoon the crumble mixture over the rhubarb and bake for 15 minutes.

Spicy Berries with Vanilla Yoghurt *Serves 6*

The chilli and herb infusion gives these berries a very interesting flavour.

Ingredients

1 cup water

¼ cup maple syrup

vanilla pod, split with seeds scraped out (reserve the seeds for another use)

½ cup mint leaves roughly chopped

¼ cup basil leaves, roughly chopped

¼ teaspoon ground chilli

350 g mixed berries

200 g fresh strawberries, washed and hulled

½ teaspoon vanilla essence

200 g low-fat natural yoghurt

Method

1. Heat the water in a pan with the maple syrup and vanilla pod and bring to the boil.
2. Place the herbs in a piece of muslin and tie around with string to make a bag. Drop the bag into the water with the chilli.
3. Set aside to cool to room temperature.
4. Pour the liquid over the mixed berries and refrigerate for at least 2 hours.
5. Add the strawberries approximately 1 hour before serving.
6. Stir the vanilla essence through the yoghurt and serve with the berries.

Frozen berries

While we should aim to eat seasonally 99 per cent of the time, some foods are so good for us they're worth eating all year round. Cranberries are grown almost exclusively in North America, but are available frozen. Raspberries, blueberries and blackberries also freeze well and are a much cheaper alternative once the Australian growing season has passed.

Yoghurt, Pistachio and Fig Cakes *Serves 4-6*

Most of us were brought up to believe that all sweet food is a treat so it's hard to deny ourselves that pleasure from time to time. The compromise may be to make healthy sweet treats and enjoy them more often than not.

Ingredients

5 dried figs, chopped
2 tablespoons rose water
3 large free range eggs
½ cup honey
350 g low-fat yoghurt
zest of 1 lemon and ½ orange
juice of ½ lemon
¼ cup coarse semolina
30 g pistachios roughly chopped

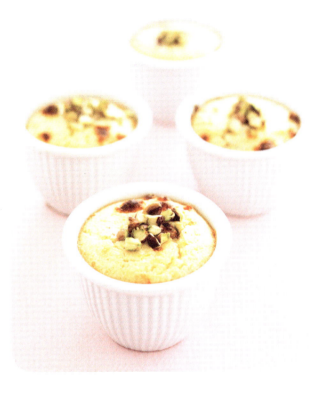

Method

1. Preheat the oven to 180°C and place a baking tray with boiling water in the oven to stay hot.
2. Soak the figs in rosewater for 15 minutes.
3. Separate the eggs and combine the honey with the egg yolks in a bowl.
4. To the egg yolk mixture, add the yoghurt, lemon and orange zest, lemon juice, figs and semolina and combine well.
5. In a separate bowl, whisk the egg whites until stiff peaks form. Fold the egg yolk mixture into the egg whites.
6. Sprinkle a spoon of chopped pistachios into the bottom of individual greased ramekin dishes.
7. Spoon the yoghurt mixture into each dish.
8. Place the ramekins into the baking tray (the water should come halfway up the sides of each dish).
9. Bake for 20 minutes or until the top of the sponge is light golden on top.

Healthier Anzacs *Makes approx 12 biscuits*

Healthier or not, these are still high in energy and should be enjoyed in moderation.

Ingredients

1 cup rolled oats
¾ cup wholemeal spelt flour
1 pinch sea salt
¼ cup grapeseed oil
3 tablespoons rice syrup
1 tablespoon boiling water
1 teaspoon low-allergy baking powder

Method

1. Preheat the oven to 190°C.
2. Put the oats into a mixing bowl with the flour and the salt.
3. In a small pan heat the oil and rice syrup together.
4. In a separate small bowl, add the boiling water to the baking powder.
5. Pour the baking powder and water into the oil and syrup and stir continually while it fizzes up and the liquids combine.
6. Mix the wet ingredients into the dry and combine until the mix forms a ball.
7. Roll the biscuit mixture using a rolling pin on a floured bench (or rolling sheet). Cut the biscuits using a biscuit cutter.
8. Bake in the oven for 10 minutes.

Baking powder

Most modern baking powders contain high temperature aluminium salts such as calcium aluminium phosphate. Aluminium in excess is detrimental to our health and has been associated with Alzheimer's disease. While the amounts present in a teaspoon or so of baking powder may not do any harm, you can use a low-allergy baking powder containing neither aluminium nor gluten.

Honey and Linseed Biscuits *Makes 24 cookies*

These biscuits are made using two 5-star performing fats—tahini (made from sesame seeds) and linseeds (flaxseeds)—making them immeasurably better than shop-bought biscuits likely to contain trans and saturated fats. They don't contain flour, making them ideal for those on wheat-free diets. If you have a gluten intolerance, you can substitute millet flakes for the oats.

Ingredients

½ cup tahini
½ cup honey
1½ cups rolled oats
½ cup linseeds (flaxseeds)
1 teaspoon ground cinnamon

Method

1. Preheat oven to 180°C.
2. Mix all ingredients together.
3. Place golf ball sized portions on lined tray. Press flat with a fork, leaving plenty of room as cookies will spread.
4. Cook for 20 minutes or until lightly golden.
5. Allow to cool on tray for 5–10 minutes as cookies will be soft.
6. Remove when firm and place on a wire rack to cool.

Note: Like nuts, linseeds should always be stored in the refrigerator. They are available from health food stores and are either brown or golden. Golden linseeds have a higher protein content than brown but have fewer omega-3 fats.

Carrot and Pumpkin Tea Loaf *Serves 8*

This loaf is a great source of antioxidants and sweet enough to be an enjoyable treat for your kids' play snack, but not too sweet to send them into a sugar-crazed frenzy. With the oil and mashed pumpkin, it will always be moist so don't make the mistake of thinking it's uncooked.

Ingredients

½ cup camellia tea oil
2 free range eggs
¼ cup honey
1 carrot, finely grated
1 cup mashed pumpkin
1 cup self-raising wholemeal flour
½ cup walnuts, chopped
½ teaspoon cinnamon
½ teaspoon mixed spice

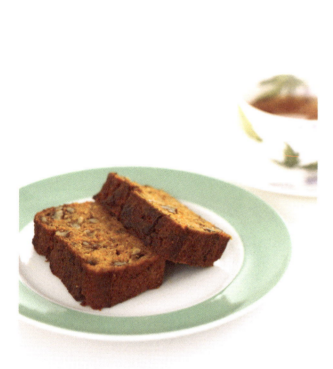

Method

1. Preheat the oven to 180°C.
2. Lightly oil a loaf tin and line the base with baking paper.
3. Mix the oil, eggs and honey until well combined. Add the remaining ingredients and mix well.
4. Fill the loaf tin and bake for 55–60 minutes.
5. Set aside to cool before turning out onto a wire rack to cool.

Bittersweet Orange Chocolate and Pomegranate *Serves 4*

The combination of pomegranate and orange with rosewater and dark chocolate is delicious. This dish can be made in advance of your guests arriving and it's extremely good for you.

Ingredients

3 oranges
1 pomegranate
½ bunch chopped mint
¼ cup rosewater
1 teaspoon pomegranate molasses
35 g dark chocolate

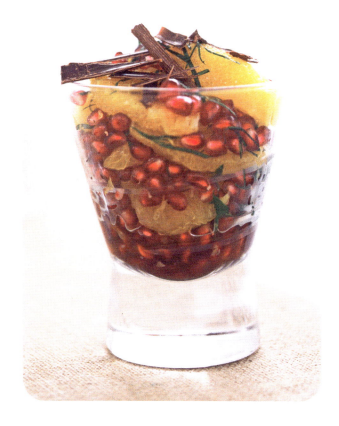

Tip: *To remove seeds from a pomegranate, lightly score the skin from top to bottom. Peel back the skin, and remove the seeds from the bitter membrane with your fingers.*

Method

1. Remove the peel and pith from the oranges and divide into segments.
2. Remove the seeds from the pomegranate and mix the two fruits together in a bowl.
3. Add the mint.
4. Combine the rosewater with the pomegranate molasses and pour over the fruit and mint. Serve in individual dishes with a few dark chocolate shavings over the top of each.

Baked Persimmon Stuffed with Cashews and Apricot

The mild flavour of persimmons contrasted with the sharp apricot is perfect in these baked persimmons. We suggest you serve this dessert after quite a light main meal and use small fruits as the dish is quite filling.

Ingredients

¼ cup raw cashews, roasted and chopped
6 dried apricot halves, cut into small pieces
2 tablespoons cashew nut spread
4 firm persimmons
low-fat yoghurt, to serve

Method

1. Preheat the oven to 180°C.
2. Combine the roasted cashews, apricots and nut spread into a paste.
3. Cut the stalks off the persimmons and, using an apple corer, remove the centre from each persimmon.
4. Stuff the cashew and apricot paste into the centre of the persimmons.
5. Cover each individually with foil and place in a baking tray filled with 3 cm of water. Bake in the oven for 25–30 minutes.
6. Serve with low-fat natural yoghurt.

Note: Select persimmons with a green cap that are free from bruises and firm to touch. Ripe persimmons range in colour from pale orange, to deep red–orange, depending upon the time of season and the variety. They will keep out of the refrigerator for up to 5 days.

REFERENCES

Anderson JW, Johnstone BM & Cook-Newell ME, 'Meta-analysis of the effects of soy protein intake on serum lipids', *New England Journal of Medicine*, 1995, 333(5), pp 276–82.

Barzel US & Massey LK, 'Excess dietary protein can adversely affect bone', *Journal of Nutrition*, 1998, 128, pp 1051–3.

Beresford SA, Johnson KC, Ritenbaugh C et al, 'Low-fat dietary pattern and risk of colorectal cancer', *JAMA*, 2006, 295, pp 643–54.

Bidel S, Hu G, Sundvall J, Kaprio J & Tuomilehto J, 'Effects of coffee consumption on glucose tolerance, serum glucose and insulin levels—a cross-sectional analysis', *Horm Metab Res*, 2006, 38(1), pp 38–43.

Cerhan JR, Saag KG, Merlino LA, Mikuls TR & Criswell LA, 'Antioxidant micronutrients and risk of rheumatoid arthritis in a cohort of older women', *American Journal of Epidemiology*, 2003, 157(4), pp 345–54.

Choi HK, Willett WC, Stampfer MJ, Rimm E & Hu FB, 'Dairy consumption and risk of type 2 diabetes mellitus in men: a prospective study', *Archives of Internal Medicine*, 2005, 165(9), pp 997–1003.

Cordain L, Boyd Eaton S, Brand-Miller J, Mann N & Himm K, 'The paradoxical nature of hunter-gatherer diets: meat based, yet non-atherogenic', *European Journal of Clinical Nutrition*, 2002, 56, Suppl 1, pp S42–52.

Cordain L, Boyd Eaton S, Sebastian A, Mann N, Lindeberg S, Watkins BA, O'Keefe JH & Brand-Miller J, 'Origins and evolution of the Western diet: health implications for the 21st century', *American Journal of Clinical Nutrition*, 2005, 81, pp 341–54.

Covas MI, Nyyssonen K, Poulsen HE et al, 'The effect of polyphenols in olive oil on heart disease risk factors: a randomized trial', *Annals of Internal Medicine*, 2006, 145(5), pp 333–41.

Denke MA, Adams-Huet B & Nguyen AT, 'Individual cholesterol variation in response to a margarine- or butter-based diet: a study in families', *JAMA*, 2000, 284(21), pp 2740–7.

Douglas RM, Hemila H, D'Souza R, Chalker EB & Treacy B, 'Vitamin C for preventing and treating the common cold', *Cochrane Database Syst Rev*, 2004, Oct 18, (4), CD000980.

Dubost J et al (2005) 'Identification and qualification of ergothioneine in cultivated mushrooms by liquid chromatography mass spectroscopy'. 230th American Chemical Society, 2005, Washington DC.

Fenoll J, Hellin P, Martinez CM & Flores P, 'Pesticide residue analysis of vegetables by gas chromatography with electron-capture detection', *J AOAC Int*, 2007, 90(1), pp 263–70.

Foster-Powell K, Holt S & Brand-Miller J, 'International table of glycemic index and glycemic load values', *American Journal of Clinical Nutrition*, 2002, 76(1), pp 5–56.

Fraser GE, Sabate J, Beeson WL & Strahan TM, 'A possible protective effect of nut consumption on risk of coronary heart disease' The Adventist Health Study, *Archives of Internal Medicine*, 1992, 152(7), pp 1416–24.

Genkinger JM, Hunter DJ, Spiegelman D et al, 'Dairy products and ovarian cancer: a pooled analysis of 12 cohort studies', *Cancer Epidemiology Biomarkers and Prevention*, 2006, 15(2), pp 364–72.

Giovannucci E, 'Tomatoes, tomato-based products, lycopene, and cancer: review of the epidemiologic literature', *Journal of the National Cancer Institute*, 1999, Feb 17, 91(4), pp 317–31.

Giovannucci E, Liu Y, Platz EA, Stampfer MJ & Willett WC, 'Risk factors for prostate cancer incidence and progression in the health professionals follow-up study', *International Journal of Cancer*, 2007, Apr 20 (Epub).

GISSI-Prevenzione Investigators, 'Dietary supplementation with n-3 polyunsaturated fatty acids and vitamin E after myocardial infarction: results of the GISSI-Prevenzione trial', *The Lancet*, 1999, 354, pp 447–55.

Halton TL & Hu F, 'The effects of high protein diets on thermogenesis, satiety and weight loss: a critical review', *Journal of the American College of Nutrition*, 2004, 23(5), pp 373–85.

Han DH, Lee MJ & Kin JH, 'Antioxidant and apoptosis-inducing activities of ellagic acid', *Anticancer Research*, 2006, 26(5A), pp 3601–6.

Hernán MA, Takkouche B, Caamaño-Isorna F & Gestal-Otero JJ, 'A meta-analysis of coffee drinking, cigarette smoking and the risk of Parkinson's disease', *Annals of Neurology*, 2002, 52, pp 276–84.

Hill A, Buckley JD, Murphy KJ & Howe PRC, 'Combining fish-oil supplements with regular aerobic exercise improves body composition and cardiovascular disease risk factors', *American Journal of Clinical Nutrition*, 2007, 85, pp 1267–74.

Howard BV, Manson JE, Stefanick ML et al, 'Low-fat dietary pattern and weight change over 7 years', *JAMA*, 2006a, 295(1), pp 39–49.

Howard BV, Van Horn L, Hsia J et al, 'Low-fat dietary pattern and risk of cardiovascular disease', *JAMA*, 2006b, 295, pp 655–66.

Jauhiainen T & Korpela R, 'Milk peptides and blood pressure', *Journal of Nutrition*, 2007, 137(3 Suppl 2), 825S–9S.

Johnson-Kozlow M, Fritz-Silverstein D, Barrett-Connor F & Morton D, 'Coffee consumption and cognitive function among older adults', *American Journal of Epidemiology*, 2002, 156, pp 842–50.

Krieger JW, Sitren HS, Daniels MJ & Langkamp-Henken B, 'Effects of variation in protein and carbohydrate intake on body mass and composition during energy restriction: a meta-regression', *American Journal of Clinical Nutrition*, 2006, 83, pp 260–74.

Lagiou P, Sandin S, Weiderpass E, Lagiou A, Mucci L, Trichopoulos D, Adami HO, 'Low carbohydrate-high protein diet and mortality in a cohort of Swedish women', *Journal of Internal Medicine*, 2007, 261(4), pp 366–74.

Larsson SC & Wolk A, 'Meat consumption and risk of colorectal cancer: a meta-analysis of prospective studies', *International Journal of Cancer*, 2006, 119(11), pp 2657–64.

Liebermann HR, 'Caffeine', in Smith AP & Jones DM (Eds), *Handbook of Human Performance*, vol 2, Academic Press, London, 1992, pp 49–72.

Lindsay J, Laurin D, Verreault R et al, 'Risk factors for Alzheimer's Disease: A prospective analysis from the Canadian Study of Health and Aging', *American Journal of Epidemiology*, 2002, 156, pp 445–53.

Lui S, Choi HK, Ford E, Song Y, Klevak A, Buring JE & Manson JE, 'A prospective study of dairy intake and the risk of type 2 diabetes in women', *Diabetes Care*, 2006, 29(7), pp 1579–84.

Maia L & de Mendonca A, 'Does caffeine intake protect from Alzheimer's disease?', *European Journal of Neurology*, 2002, 9, pp 377–82.

Mannisto S, Smith-Warner SA, Spiegelman D et al, 'Dietary carotenoids and risk of lung cancer in a pooled analysis of seven cohort studies', *Cancer Epidemiology Biomarkers & Prevention*, 2004, 13(1), pp 40–8.

Nichols PD, Virtue P, Mooney BD, Elliot NG & Yearsley GK, 'Seafood the Good Food. The oil (fat) content and composition of Australian commercial fishes, shellfishes and crustaceans', CSIRO Marine Research, 1998.

Omenn GS, Goodman GE, Thornquist MD, Balmes J, Cullen MR, Glass A, Keogh JP, Meyskens FL, Valanis B, Williams JH, Barnhart S & Hammar S, 'Effects of a combination of beta carotene and vitamin A on lung cancer and cardiovascular disease', *New England Journal of Medicine*, 1996, 334(18), pp 1150–5.

Pagano R, Negri E, Decarli A & La Vecchia C, 'Coffee drinking and prevalence of bronchial asthma', *Chest*, 1988, 94, pp 386–9.

Prentice RL, Caan B, Chlebowski RT et al, 'Low-fat dietary pattern and risk of invasive breast cancer', *JAMA*, 2006, 295, pp 629–42.

Ratcliffe B, Collins AR, Glass HJ, Hillman K & Kemble RJT, 'The effect of cooking on the protective effect of broccoli against damage to DNA in colonocytes', in Johnson IT & Fenwick GR, *Dietary Anticarcinogens and Antimutagens: Chemical and Biological Aspects*, Cambridge, Royal Society of Chemistry, 2000, pp 161–4.

Sacks FM, Lichtenstein A, Van Horn L, Harris W, Kris-Etherton P, Winston M, American Heart Association Nutrition Committee, 'Soy protein, isoflavones, and cardiovascular health: an American Heart Association Science Advisory for professionals from the Nutrition Committee', *Circulation*, 2006, 113(7), pp 1034–44.

Schwartz J & Weiss ST, 'Caffeine intake and asthma symptoms', *Annals of Epidemiology*, 1992, 2(5), pp 627–35.

Simopoulos AP & Salem N Jr, 'n-3 fatty acids in eggs from range-fed Greek chickens', *New England Journal of Medicine*, 1989, 321(20), p 1412.

Strom BL, Schinnar R, Ziegler EE, Barnhart KT, Sammel MD, Macones GA, Stallings VA, Drulis JM, Nelson SE & Hanson SA, 'Exposure to soy-based formula in infancy and endocrinological and reproductive outcomes in young adulthood', *JAMA*, 2001, 286(7), pp 807–14.

Tavani A & La Vecchia C, 'Coffee and cancer: a review of epidemiological studies 1990–1999', *European Journal of Cancer Prevention*, 2000, 9, pp 241–56.

The -tocopherol -Carotene Cancer Prevention Study Group, 'The effect of vitamin E and -carotene on the incidence of lung cancer and other cancers in male smokers', *New England Journal of Medicine*, 1994, 330, pp 1029–35.

Trichopoulou A, Psaltopoulou T, Orfanos P, Hsieh C-C & Trichopoulos D, 'Low-carbohydrate-high-protein diet and long-term survival in a general population cohort', *European Journal of Clinical Nutrition*, 2007, 61, pp 575–81.

van Dam RM, Willett WC, Manson JE & Hu FB, 'Coffee, caffeine, and risk of type 2 diabetes: a prospective cohort study in younger and middle-aged US women', *Diabetes Care*, 2006, 29, pp 398–403.

Woodford K. 2007. *The Devil in the Milk*. Craig Potton Publishing, New Zealand.

Zemel MB, 'The role of dairy foods in weight management', *Journal of the American College of Nutrition*, 2005, 24(6 Suppl), pp 537S–46S.

INDEX

Reference to recipes are in *italics*

5-star performers 12
  carbohydrates 65–73
  fats 117–121
  fruit 38–46
  proteins 85–101
  vegetables 22–31

A
A2 milk 96
agricultural age 60
alcohol 129–30
allergies to milk 97
almond oil 115, 122
Alzheimer's disease 132
amino acids 82–83
animal foods, *see* meat
anthocyanins 23, 40, 45
anti-inflammatory effect of fats 108
antibacterial properties of garlic 29
antibiotics in chicken production 85
antioxidants
  in coffee 133
  in nuts and seeds 118
  in onion family 29
  in organic foods 6
  in tomatoes 30
Anzac biscuits 137, 214
apples 49, 51
apricots 39, 48, 51
Asian greens 32
Asian salad 162
asparagus 22, 32, 158
asthma, coffee and 132–33
Australian dietary recommendations 18
avocado 39–40, 48, 153, 165
Avocado gazpacho 153
Avocado mango and pine nut salad 165
avocado oil 115, 117, 122

B
bad fats 107, 111
bagels 77
Baked kingfish and mushrooms 202
Baked ling with eggplant, capsicum and lima beans 197
Baked persimmon stuffed with cashews and apricot 218
baking powder 214

bamboo shoots 35
banana bread 136
bananas 49
Barbecued chicken with preserved lemon 192
Barbecued corn with lemon infused olive oil 178
barley 65, 178, 194
Barley and Pea Risotto with Chargrilled Salmon 194
Basic tomato and basil sauce 173
basmati rice 76
bean sprouts 34
beans 65–66
beef 183, 184, 185
beetroot 35
berries 40, 48
  frozen berries 212
  recipes 149, 180, 212
beta-carotene 24, 26, 31
beta-crypytoxanthin 42
beta-sitoserol 40
'Better than mash' barley and bean pot 178
bhuja mix 136
biscotti 136
biscuits 77, 125, 136–38, 214, 215
Bittersweet orange chocolate and pomegranate 217
boiled sweets 138
bowel health 53–55, 61
brain development 108, *see also* cognitive performance
bran 55, 76
Brazil nuts 122
breads 67–68
breakfast cereals 76, 77
Breakfast quinoa 150
breakfast recipes 145–51
broad beans 76
broccoli 22, 32, 209
broccolini 32
brown rice 76
brussels sprouts 32, 181
Brussels sprouts with roasted pine nut and lemon mustard dressing 181
buckwheat 68, 151
Buckwheat pancakes with blueberry sauce and bush honey yoghurt 151
bulgur 68
burgers 103
butter 111–12, 124
butternut squash 34

C
cabbage family 22–23, 32, 34
caffeic acid 31
caffeine 131
cakes 77, 125, 136–38, 213
calcium 94
camellia tea oil 115, 117
cancer, soy products and 100
canned fruit 49
canola oil 115, 124
capsaicin 24
capsicums 24, 32
carbohydrates 52–77
cardiovascular disease 99–100, 108
CAROT trial 26
Carrot and pumpkin tea loaf 216
carrots 34, 136, 216
cashew nuts 122
catechins 131
cauliflower 34
celeriac 35
celery 35
Chachouka 148
chapatti 76
Chargrilled kangaroo steaks with hummus, silverbeet and beetroot and apple relish 189
Chargrilled salmon with asparagus, lemon and anchovy 201
Chargrilled sesame octopus and watercress salad 168
cheese 102–3, 113, 167
cheesecake 138
cherries 49
chicken 85–86, 102–3
  recipes 171, 190, 191, 192
Chicken and pomegranate salad 171
Chicken and tomato bake 191
chicory 35
chiko rolls 138
chillies 24, 32
Chilli beef and beans 183
chips 137, 138
chlorogenic acid 31, 44
chocolate 136–38
citrus fruit 40–42, 48
cocoa 128
coconut oil 115, 122–23
coffee 129–30, 132–33
cognitive performance 53, 132, *see also* brain development
colon cancer 61
complementary proteins 83

cooking 114–15, 142–44
cordial 130
corn 68–69, 178
corn oil 115, 124
coumarin 42
couscous 76
Cracked sweet and sour freekeh 179
cranberries 51
crispbreads 77
croissants 77
crumpets 77
cucumber 35, 159
Cucumber, eggplant, avocado and bulgur timbale 159
cured meats 103
curly kale 32
currants 51
cynarin 26

D
dairy foods 94–98, 102, 124
dates 51
desserts 138
dhal 177
diabetes, coffee and 133
diet
  common problems 139–41
  hunter-gatherer diets 63
  meaning of 5
  optimal human 60–61
  quick quiz 14–15
dinner recipes 182–210
doongara rice 76
doughnuts 77, 125, 138
dried fruit 51, 136
drinks 126–33
duck 103

E
eggplant 35
eggs 86–89, 102, 158, 210
ellagic acid 40, 45
endive 32
energy drinks 130
energy from protein 80
energy needs 61
ergothioneine 28
eritadenine 28
eschallots 29
exercise, carbohydrates and 53–54
Eye fillet with salsa verde 185
eye protection 108

F
Fatoush 164
fats 104–25
fennel 34
ferulic acid 31

fibre, *see also* soluble fibre
  bowel health and 54–55
  in avocado 39
  in capsicums and chillies 24
  in citrus fruit 42
  in kiwi fruit 44
  in vegetables and fruit 18
  insoluble fibre 23
figs 51
fish 89–90, 102
  dietary recommendations 110
  oily fish 89, 120, 122
  recipes 156, 170, 193–203
five-star performers 12
flavonoids 42
flavoured milk 130
flavoured water 130
flax seed oil 115, 119, 122
folate
  in avocado 39
  in cabbage family 23
  in citrus fruit 42
  in globe artichokes 26
  in green leafy vegetables 24
food pyramids 10–15, 140–41
FOS 29
free range chicken 85–86
freekeh 70–71, 161, 179
freezing vegetables and fruit 18, 212
friands 136
fructo-oligosaccharides 29
fruit 10, 16–18, 60
fruit bars 136
fruit bread 136
fruit juice 129
fruit pies 137
fruitcake 136

G
game meats 91, 102, 169, 188, 189
game of great health 11
garlic 33, 179
Garlic and chickpea mash 179
ginger 34
globe artichokes 26, 33
glucose 53
glutathione 40
glycaemic index 18, 56–59, 80
good fats 107–8, 111
good performers 12
goose 103
grain, processing of 56–58
grape seed oil 115, 123
grapefruit 48
grapes 49
green beans 34
green leafy vegetables 24–26, 155, 176
green peas 29–30

Green salad with avocado, almond and mustard dressing 166
Green tea barley risotto with mushrooms and asparagus 208
Grilled blue eye cod with sage, lentils and roast capsicum 199
Grilled chicken with smoked paprika, chilli and capsicum sauce 190
Grilled goat cheese, hazelnut and cranberry salad 167
Grilled snapper fillet with bulgur, parsley and roasted almonds 195
guava 42, 48

H
hazelnut oil 115
hazelnuts 122
Healthier anzacs 214
Healthy harira 187
heart disease 99–100, 108
high-fibre foods 55
high protein diets 78
honey 62–63, 215
Honey and linseed biscuits 215
honeydew melon 49
hot chocolate 130
hunter-gatherer diets 63

I
ice cream 137, 138
immune system 108
insoluble fibre 23
insulin resistance 58
iron requirements 81
isoflavones 99–100

J
Japanese diet 105
jelly 138
juices 128

K
kaempferol 40
Kangaroo fillets with macadamia and plum sauce 188
Kangaroo Thai salad 169
Kingfish with pine nuts and cucumber and lemon salsa 203
kitchen items 143
kiwi fruit 44, 48
kumquat 48

L
lactose intolerance 97
lamb recipes 186, 187
lard 125

lean pork 93
legumes 65–66, 102, 179, *see also names of legumes*
Lentil and freekeh patties with coleslaw 161
Lentil dhal 177
lentils 65–66, 161, 177
lentinan 28
liabilities 13
Light meals and entrees 152–61
Lime, corn and coriander salsa 174
limonene 42
linseed (flax seed) oil 115, 119, 122
liquorice 137
liver 92–93, 102
lobster 90
longer chain fats 82
lutein
　in cabbage family 23
　in green leafy vegetables 24–26
　in kiwi fruit 44
　in tomatoes 31
luteolin 26
lychees 49
lycopene 30

M
macadamia oil 115
macadamias 123
magnesium 40
mangoes 48, 51
maple syrup 63
margarines 111–12, 124
Marinated lamb and vegetable kebabs 186
marrow 34
mayonnaise 123, 125
meat
　case for eating 81–82
　comparisons of 92
　fat content 125
　in early human diet 60–61
　recipes 182–92
　red meat 93, 102–3
Mediterranean diet 105
Mediterranean mackerel with basil and rocket pesto 196
Mediterranean mussels 160
menopause 100–101
mercury in fish 90
milk 6, 94–98, 103, 129–30
millet 76
mineral water 128
minerals 18
mixed grain fruit bread 76
mountain bread 76
muesli 71–72, 146
muesli bars 136–37

muffins 76–77, 136–37
mung bean noodles 76
mushrooms 28, 33, 154
mussels 90

N
naringin 42
nectarines 49
nobelitin 42
noodles 76
nougat 138
nuts 118–19, 124, 136–37
　nut spreads 122
　recipes 152, 175, 213

O
oatcakes 76
oats 71–72, 147
offal 61, 92–93
oils 114–15, *see also* fats
oily fish 89, 120, 122
okra 34
Olive, coriander, tomato, chilli and lime salsa 172
olive oil 115, 120–21, 122
omega-3 fats 88, 106–10
onion family 29, 33
online shopping 18
oranges 48, 217
organic foods 6, 86
oysters 90, 98, 157
Oysters with diced vegetables and herb vinaigrette 157

P
palm oil 125
pancakes 137–38, 151
papaya 44, 48
pappadams 77
Parkinson's disease 132
parsley 33
parsnips 35
party pies 138
passionfruit 44, 48
pasta 73, 76
pastries 125, 138
peaches 49, 51
peanut oil 115, 123
peanuts 123
pears 49, 51
peas 29–30, 33
pecans 122
persimmons 45, 48, 218
phenol compounds 120
phytates 55
phytochemicals 23
pikelets 77
pine nuts 122
pineapple 49
pistachios 122

pita bread 76
plant sterol margarines 124
player profiles
　carbohydrates 75
　dried fruit 51
　fats 122–23
　fresh fruit 48–49
　proteins 102–3
　vegetables 32–33
plums 49
Poached eggs with asparagus and shaved goat cheese 158
Poached ocean trout with green tea salsa 200
polenta 77
polyphenols 131
polyunsaturated fats 106, 125
pomegranates 45–46, 48
popcorn 136
pork 93, 102
porridge 77, 147
potassium 23, 40
potatoes 35, 77
prawns 102
pretzels 137
processed grain 56–58
protein 78–103
protein bars 138
prunes 51
puffed grains 77
pulses 65–67, 102, *see also names of pulses*
pumpernickel bread 67
pumpkin 34, 207, 216

Q
quick quiz 14–15
quinoa 72, 150, 163
Quinoa tabbouleh 163

R
radish 35
raisins 51, 137
rankings
　carbohydrates 64
　drinks 126–27
　fats 116
　fruit 37–51
　proteins 84
　treats 136–38
　vegetables 20–21
red cabbage 32, 180
red meat 93, 102, 103, *see also* meat
refined oils 124
reproductive health 101
reserves 13
rhubarb 49, 211
Rhubarb and ginger nut crumble 211

Index　223

rice 76–77, 194, 208
rice bran oil 124
rice crackers 77
rice noodles 77
rocket 33
rockmelon 46, 48
Rolled beef with asparagus and shallots 184
rooibos tea 128, 131
Ruby red ocean trout 198
runner beans 34
rutin 22
rye bread 68

S

safflower oil 115, 123
salad dressing 125
salads 162–71
salami 103
Salmon and cannelini bean salad 170
salsas and sauces 172–75
sandwiches 18
saponins 22
Sardine, avocado and capsicum grill 156
sausage rolls 138
sausages 103
Sautéed silverbeet, olive and fennel pasta 206
scones 137
seafood 98, 102, 122, *see also* fish recipes 157, 160, 168
sedentary lifestyles 58
seeds 118–19, *see also* grain; legumes; pulses
semolina 76
sesame oil 115, 123
sesame seeds 122
shallots 29
Shiitake and buckwheat soup 154
shopping 144
shortening 125
side dishes 176–81
side salads 18
silverbeet 33, 206, 207, 210
Silverbeet, pumpkin and pine nut roll 207
Silverbeet, ricotta and vegetable frittata 210
skim milk 129
smoothies 129
snow peas 29–30

soba noodles 76
soda water 128
soft drinks 130
soluble fibre 55
soups and stews 153, 177, 178
sourdough bread 76
soy products 99–102
  soy chips 137
  soy oil 115, 124
  tofu 209
Spicy berries with vanilla yoghurt 212
Spicy red cabbage with cranberries 180
Spicy roast nuts 152
spinach 33
spring onion 29
Spring veggie pie 204–5
sprouts 34
squid 102
Stir-fried Asian greens 176
stoneground bread 67
Strawberry breakfast trifle 149
suet 125
sugar snap peas 29–30
sugars 62
sulphur 29
sultanas 51
summer squash 34
sunflower oil 115, 123
sunflower seeds 122
swedes 35
sweet potatoes 34
sweet recipes 149, 211–18
sweetcorn 68–69, 178
Swiss chard 33

T

tabbouleh 163
tahini 122
tallow 125
tangeretin 42
tannins 40, 45
taro 35
taste of vegetables and fruit 18
taurine 82
tea 128, 131
textured vegetable protein 103
timbale 159
tisanes 131
toffee 138
Tofu, broccoli and sesame stir fry 209
tomatoes 30–31, 33, 148, 173, 191

tortilla 76
trans fats 106
treats 10–11, 134–38
Triple grain muesli 146
turkey 85–86, 102
turnips 35
TVP 103

V

veal 103
vegetable juices 128, 130
vegetables 16–36
  in early human diet 60
  in food pyramid 10
vegetarian recipes 155, 204–10
Vegetarian san choy bau 155
vitamins 18
  vitamin A 82
  vitamin B6: 22
  vitamin B12 requirements 81–82
  vitamin C 23–24, 39, 40
  vitamin E 39
  vitamin K 23, 26, 40

W

walnut oil 115
Walnut pesto 175
walnuts 122, 175
water 128
watercress 33, 34
watermelon 49
weight control 18
what to eat 7
white bread 77
white rice 77
whole grain bread 68
wholemeal bread 77
wholemeal pasta 73
why some foods are better than others 7
winter squash 34

Y

yams 35
yoghurt 94–98, 102–3, 213
Yoghurt, pistachio and fig cakes 213

Z

zeaxanthin 24–26, 31
zinc requirements 81
zucchini 34